Jon Pynoos, PhD
Penny Hollander Feldman, PhD
Joann Ahrens, MPA
Editors

Linking Housing and Services for Older Adults: Obstacles, Options, and Opportunities

Linking Housing and Services for Older Adults: Obstacles, Options, and Opportunities has been co-published simultaneously as *Journal of Housing for the Elderly*, Volume 18, Numbers 3/4 2004.

Pre-publication
REVIEWS,
COMMENTARIES,
EVALUATIONS . . .

"This book is AN INVALUABLE RESOURCE FOR STUDENTS, RESEARCHERS, POLICYMAKERS, AND ACADEMICS interested in housing and supportive services for older adults."

Victoria Cotrell, PhD
Assistant Professor
Graduate School of Social Work
Portland State University

The Haworth Press, Inc.
New York

Linking Housing and Services for Older Adults: Obstacles, Options, and Opportunities

Linking Housing and Services for Older Adults: Obstacles, Options, and Opportunities has been co-published simultaneously as *Journal of Housing for the Elderly*, Volume 18, Numbers 3/4 2004.

The *Journal of Housing for the Elderly*™ Monographic "Separates"

Below is a list of "separates," which in serials librarianship means a special issue simultaneously published as a special journal issue or double-issue *and* as a "separate" hardbound monograph. (This is a format which we also call a "DocuSerial.")

"Separates" are published because specialized libraries or professionals may wish to purchase a specific thematic issue by itself in a format which can be separately cataloged and shelved, as opposed to purchasing the journal on an on-going basis. Faculty members may also more easily consider a "separate" for classroom adoption.

"Separates" are carefully classified separately with the major book jobbers so that the journal tie-in can be noted on new book order slips to avoid duplicate purchasing.

You may wish to visit Haworth's website at . . .

http://www.HaworthPress.com

. . . to search our online catalog for complete tables of contents of these separates and related publications.

You may also call 1-800-HAWORTH (outside US/Canada: 607-722-5857), or Fax 1-800-895-0582 (outside US/Canada: 607-771-0012), or e-mail at:

docdelivery@haworthpress.com

Linking Housing and Services for Older Adults: Obstacles, Options, and Opportunities, edited by Jon Pynoos, PhD, Penny Hollander Feldman, PhD, and Joann Ahrens, MPA (Vol. 18, No. 3/4, 2004). *In-depth examination from a cross-section of experts about the advantages and problems of linking housing with supportive services for the aging.*

Physical Environments and Aging: Critical Contributions of M. Powell Lawton to Theory and Practice, edited by Rick J. Scheidt, PhD, and Paul G. Windley (Vol. 17, No. 1/2, 2003). *"Excellent. . . . Thoughtful. . . . Outstanding. . . . Will bring the reader up to date in many ways. So much of Lawton's work in environment and aging is reflected in this comprehensive book. It honors Lawton not only through a discussion of his theoretic and substantive contributions, but also through its warm memories of him. Dr. Lawton helped so many students and colleagues in so many ways. His important legacy clearly lives on." (Robert L. Rubinstein, PhD, Professor, Gerontology Doctoral Program, University of Maryland-Baltimore County; Co-author,* Old Souls: Aged Women, Poverty, and the Experience of God)

Assisted Living: Sobering Realities, edited by Benyamin Schwarz, PhD (Vol. 15, No. 1/2, 2001). *Explores the implications of the current state of one of the fastest-growing areas in housing for the elderly.*

Housing Choices and Well-Being of Older Adults: Proper Fit, edited by Leon A. Pastalan, PhD, and Benyamin Schwarz, PhD (Vol. 14, No. 1/2, 2001). *"Convincing . . . Helpful in improving accessibility. . . . With this collaborative work we are one step closer to taming fears, domesticating dreams, and realizing gerontopia." (Ruth S. Brent, PhD, Professor and Chair, Department of Environmental Design, University of Missouri-Columbia)*

Making Aging in Place Work, edited by Leon A. Pastalan, PhD (Vol. 13, No. 1/2, 1999). *Addressing issues ranging from home modification to treatment of depression, this book will help you identify the needs of the elderly in order to offer them a comfortable and more independent life.*

Shelter and Service Issues for Aging Populations: International Perspectives, edited by Leon A. Pastalan, PhD (Vol. 12, No. 1/2, 1997). *"Provides an international perspective on meeting the housing and service needs of the elderly. The book outlines the strengths and weaknesses of different approaches, policies, and cost-effective, successful arrangements." (Older Americans Report)*

Housing Decisions for the Elderly: To Move or Not to Move, edited by Leon Pastalan, PhD (Vol. 11, No. 2, 1995). *"This insightful book thoroughly explores the crucial decisions many elderly face, and it provides a comprehensive overview of the complex problems that are associated with these decisions." (Benyamin Schwarz, PhD, Assistant Professor, Environmental Design Department, University of Missouri)*

University-Linked Retirement Communities: Student Visions of Eldercare, edited by Leon A. Pastalan, PhD, and Benyamin Schwarz (Vol. 11, No. 1, 1994). *"A masterpiece. . . . Provides one of the most comprehensive sets of illustrations for integrating research-based theory with design to date. . . . The contribution this book makes to a better understanding of the multidisciplinary nature of the design process is profound."(Ronald G. Phillips, ArchD, Director, Graduate Studies Program, Department of Environmental Design, University of Missouri-Columbia)*

Congregate Housing for the Elderly: Theoretical, Policy, and Programmatic Perspectives, edited by Lenard W. Kaye, DSW, and Abraham Monk, PhD (Vol. 9, No. 1/2, 1992). *"Significant authorities present concise factual chapters about federal housing policies, services for elders, models of service assisted housing, enhanced or supported housing and 'assisted living,' and specifically, the federal congregate Housing Services Program." (Journal of the American Geriatrics Society)*

Residential Care Services for the Elderly: Business Guide for Home-Based Eldercare, edited by Doris K. Williams, PhD (Vol. 8, No. 2, 1991). *"A how-to-do-it manual for persons considering establishing a home-based business to provide residential care services for elderly people." (Science Books & Films)*

Housing Risks and Homelessness Among the Urban Elderly, edited by Sharon M. Keigher, PhD (Vol. 8, No. 1, 1991). *"A good beginning for an understanding of homelessness among older persons. . . . Useful for policymakers in their pursuit of useful and valid information that would serve to focus the direction of future policies and programs related to homelessness, especially among those who are older." (Educational Gerontology)*

Granny Flats as Housing for the Elderly: International Perspectives, edited by N. Michael Lazarowich, PhD (Vol. 7, No. 2, 1991). *"An informative guide to the latest experimental projects and government programs to encourage the provision of 'granny flats' or 'echo housing'– apartment or other dwelling units which are wholly or partly linked to or within a family dwelling." (Tony Warnes, Kings College, London)*

Optimizing Housing for the Elderly: Homes Not Houses, edited by Leon A. Pastalan, PhD (Vol. 7, No. 1, 1991). *"Especially helpful to planners and policy developers in the area of housing alternatives for the elderly. There is a clear effort to provide a range of options for professional intervention." (Science Books & Films)*

Aging in Place: The Role of Housing and Social Supports, edited by Leon A. Pastalan, PhD (Vol. 6, No. 1/2, 1990). *"Emphasizes the practicalities of keeping people going in independent housing." (British Journal of Psychiatry)*

The Retirement Community Movement: Some Contemporary Issues, edited by Leon Pastalan, PhD (Vol. 5, No. 2, 1989). *The practical implications of the research findings provided in this key volume help readers to identify and satisfy the needs of retirement community residents.*

Lifestyles and Housing of Older Adults: The Florida Experience, edited by Leon A. Pastalan, PhD, and Marie E. Cowart, DPH, RN (Vol. 5, No. 1, 1989). *"A good introductory source for students to understand recent efforts to amalgamate living environments and service delivery systems in order to provide better care for the elderly." (Community Alternatives)*

Aging at Home: How the Elderly Adjust Their Housing Without Moving, edited by Raymond J. Struyk, PhD, and Harold M. Katsura, MCRP (Vol. 4, No. 2, 1988). *"Of value in the development of a comprehensive theory of environmental adjustment relevant regardless of age for those for whom living in place has become problematic." (Disabilities Studies Quarterly)*

Continuing Care Retirement Communities: Political, Social, and Financial Issues, edited by Ian A. Morrison, Ruth Bennett, PhD, Susana Frisch, MA, and Barry J. Gurland, MD (Vol. 3, No. 1/2, 1986). *"Well-written and comprehensive in scope." (The Gerontologist)*

Retirement Communities: An American Original, edited by Michael E. Hunt, Allan G. Feldt, Robert W. Marans, Leon A. Pastalan, and Kathleen L. Vakalo (Vol. 1, No. 3/4, 1984). *A thorough, informative volume on retirement communities in the United States.*

Linking Housing and Services for Older Adults: Obstacles, Options, and Opportunities

Jon Pynoos, PhD
Penny Hollander Feldman, PhD
Joann Ahrens, MPA
Editors

Linking Housing and Services for Older Adults: Obstacles, Options, and Opportunities has been co-published simultaneously as *Journal of Housing for the Elderly*, Volume 18, Numbers 3/4 2004.

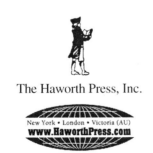

The Haworth Press, Inc.

New York • London • Victoria (AU)
www.HaworthPress.com

Linking Housing and Services for Older Adults: Obstacles, Options, and Opportunities has been co-published simultaneously as *Journal of Housing for the Elderly*™, Volume 18, Numbers 3/4 2004.

The development, preparation, and publication of this work has been undertaken with great care. However, the publisher, employees, editors, and agents of The Haworth Press and all imprints of The Haworth Press, Inc., including The Haworth Medical Press® and Pharmaceutical Products Press®, are not responsible for any errors contained herein or for consequences that may ensue from use of materials or information contained in this work. Opinions expressed by the author(s) are not necessarily those of The Haworth Press, Inc. With regard to case studies, identities and circumstances of individuals discussed herein have been changed to protect confidentiality. Any resemblance to actual persons, living or dead, is entirely coincidental.

Cover design by Deborah Huelsbergen

Library of Congress Catalog-in-Publication Data

Linking housing and services for older adults : obstacles, options, and opportunities / Jon Pynoos, Penny Hollander Feldman, Joann Ahrens, editors.
     p. cm.
     "Linking Housing and Services for Older Adults : Obstacles, Options, and Opportunities has been co-published simultaneously as Journal of Housing for the Elderly, volume 18, numbers 3/4 2004."
     Includes bibliographical references and index.
     ISBN 0-7890-2778-X (hard cover : alk. paper) – ISBN 0-7890-2779-8 (soft cover : alk. paper)
     1. Older people–Housing–Government policy–United States. 2. Older people–Services for–United States. 3. Housing subsidies–United States. 4. Public housing–United States. I. Pynoos, Jon. II. Feldman, Penny Hollander. III. Ahrens, Joann. IV. Journal of housing for the elderly.
    HD7287.92.U54L56 2005
    363.5'946'0973–dc22

                                    2004021700

Indexing, Abstracting & Website/Internet Coverage

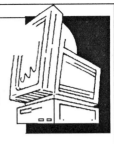

This section provides you with a list of major indexing & abstracting services and other tools for bibliographic access. That is to say, each service began covering this periodical during the year noted in the right column. Most Websites which are listed below have indicated that they will either post, disseminate, compile, archive, cite or alert their own Website users with research-based content from this work. (This list is as current as the copyright date of this publication.)

Abstracting, Website/Indexing Coverage . . . . Year When Coverage Began

- *Abstracts in Social Gerontology: Current Literature on Aging* 1983

- *AgeInfo CD-ROM* 1995

- *AgeLine Database <http://research.aarp.org/ageline>* 1983

- *AGRICOLA Database (AGRICultural OnLine Access)*
  A Bibliographic database of citations to the agricultural
  literature created by the National Agricultural Library
  and its cooperators <http://www.natl.usda.gov/ag98> 1989

- *AGRIS <http://www.fao.org/agris/>* 1989

- *Applied Social Sciences Index & Abstracts (ASSIA) (Online:*
  ASSI via Data-Star) (CDRom: ASSIA Plus)
  <http://www.csa.com> 1993

- *Architectural Periodicals Index* 1993

- *Business Source Corporate: coverage of nearly 3,350 quality*
  magazines and journals; designed to meet the diverse
  information needs of corporations; EBSCO Publishing
  <http://www.epnet.com/corporate/bsourcecorp.asp> 2003

(continued)

(continued)

*Special Bibliographic Notes related to special journal issues
(separates) and indexing/abstracting:*

- indexing/abstracting services in this list will also cover material in any "separate" that is co-published simultaneously with Haworth's special thematic journal issue or DocuSerial. Indexing/abstracting usually covers material at the article/chapter level.
- monographic co-editions are intended for either non-subscribers or libraries which intend to purchase a second copy for their circulating collections.
- monographic co-editions are reported to all jobbers/wholesalers/approval plans. The source journal is listed as the "series" to assist the prevention of duplicate purchasing in the same manner utilized for books-in-series.
- to facilitate user/access services all indexing/abstracting services are encouraged to utilize the co-indexing entry note indicated at the bottom of the first page of each article/chapter/contribution.
- this is intended to assist a library user of any reference tool (whether print, electronic, online, or CD-ROM) to locate the monographic version if the library has purchased this version but not a subscription to the source journal.
- individual articles/chapters in any Haworth publication are also available through the Haworth Document Delivery Service (HDDS).

Linking Housing and Services for Older Adults: Obstacles, Options, and Opportunities

CONTENTS

ABOUT THE EDITORS

Jon Pynoos, PhD, is the UPS Foundation Professor of Gerontology, Policy and Urban Planning at the Andrus Gerontology Center of the University of Southern California, as well as Director of the National Resource Center on Supportive Housing and Home Modifications. Dr. Pynoos has spent his career researching, writing, and advising the government and private sector concerning how to improve housing and long-term care policies and programs for the elderly. He has conducted a large number of applied research projects based on surveys, data analysis, and case studies on housing, home modification, aging in place, and long-term care. He has written and co-edited five books on housing and the elderly including *Housing the Aged: Design Directives and Policy Considerations* (with Victor Regnier) and *Housing Frail Elders: International Policies, Perspectives and Prospects* (with Phoebe Liebig).

Dr. Pynoos was a delegate to the two last White House Conferences on Aging and is currently a member of the California Commission on Aging. He is a founder of the National Home Modification Action Coalition that seeks to develop better policies, programs and practices to help older persons age in place.

Dr. Pynoos has been awarded both Guggenheim and Fulbright Fellowships. He is a Fellow of the Gerontological Society of America and is Past Chair of its Section on Social Research, Policy and Practice. Before moving to USC in 1979, Dr. Pynoos was Director of an Area Agency on Aging/Home Care Corporation in Massachusetts that provided a range of services to keep older persons out of institutional settings. He holds undergraduate, Master's and PhD degrees from Harvard University where he graduated Magna cum Laude.

Penny Hollander Feldman, PhD, is Vice President for Research and Evaluation at the Visiting Nurse Service of New York (VNSNY) and Director of the Center for Home Care Policy & Research. Prior to joining VNSNY, Dr. Feldman served on the faculties of the Kennedy School of Government and the Department of Health Policy and Management at the Harvard School of Public Health, where she continues as Visiting Lecturer. At the Center for Home Care Policy & Research, she directs projects focused on improving the quality, outcomes and cost-effectiveness of home-based care, supporting informed policy-making by long-term care decision-makers, and helping communities promote the health, well-being and independence of people with chronic illness or disability. Her most recent publication, which appeared in the June 2003 issue of the *Milbank Quarterly*, is a paper she co-authored with Robert Kane, entitled, *Strengthening research to improve the practice and management of long-term care.*

Joann Ahrens, MPA, Research Project Manager, joined the Center for Home Care Policy & Research in January 2002. Ms. Ahrens is managing a Robert Wood Johnson Foundation grant project, Information Brokering for Long-Term Care, which seeks to strengthen links between research-based data and information useful to policymakers and contribute to productive dialogue between researchers and policymakers. Ms. Ahrens is also the project manager for a large Agency for Healthcare Research and Quality (AHRQ)-sponsored project on the work environment and patient safety that is examining the relationships between the organizational work place, the nursing work force, and preventable adverse events in the home health care setting. In addition, Ms. Ahrens facilitates the Center's communication strategy through increased internal and external publications.

Ms. Ahrens is a graduate of the University of Pennsylvania and received a Master of Public Administration degree with a concentration in health finance from New York University's Wagner School. Previously, Ms. Ahrens managed a variety of strategic, financial, and policy projects for the CEO of VNSNY. Before joining VNSNY, Ms. Ahrens was a consultant at William M. Mercer.

About the Contributors

Dawn Alley, BS, is a doctoral student in the University of Southern California's Leonard David School of Gerontology and a research assistant at the National Resource Center on Supportive Housing and Home Modification. As a National Institute on Aging (NIA) predoctoral trainee, her main research interest is in the relationship between the environment and health for older adults.

Paula C. Carder is a Policy Development and Research Associate for NCB Development Corporation and an affiliate Assistant Professor at the University of Maryland, Baltimore County. She has conducted research on daily operations in assisted living facilities for several years, including a recent NIA-funded study of resident assessment practices. Her recent publications include "Consumer Discourse in Assisted Living" in the *Journals of Gerontology Social Sciences* (March 2004, with Mauro Hernandez), a chapter in *Gray Areas: Ethnographic Encounters with Nursing Home Culture* (2003, P. B. Stafford editor), and an article about the privacy needs of family visitors to Alzheimer's care facilities in the *Journal of Applied Gerontology* (2003, with Nancy Chapman).

Leonard Heumann is Professor Emeritus of Urban and Regional Planning and Psychology at the University of Illinois at Urbana-Champaign. He conducts research and teaches in all aspects of housing and community development planning, but for the past 28 years has been a social scientist conducting applied research in the management, planning and design of housing and support services for elderly persons.

He is the co-author or co-editor of the following books on aging in place, managing care responsibilities, and empowerment of the frail population: *Housing for the Elderly: Planning and Policy Formulation in Western Europe and North America* (1983); *Aging in Place with Dignity: International Solutions to Accommodate the Low Income and Frail Elderly* (1993); *Managing Care, Risk and Responsibility: The Challenge of the 21st Century as the Aging and Disabled Population Grows and Diversifies* (1997); and, *Empowering Frail Elderly People: Opportunities and Impediments in Housing, Health and Support Service Delivery* (2001). He has completed research on many of the aspects of efficiency, economy and quality of aging-in-place programs such as: "Aging in Conventional Housing: A Planner's Evaluation of the New Australian Home Based Care Management Programs" (1997).

He has studied frail senior populations seeking to move into and living in subsidized housing, both publicly owned and managed, and non-profit owned and managed. Among these studies are both the *1988 and 1999 National Survey of Section 202 Elderly Housing* (1989) (2001); *The Growing Needs of Elderly Persons Aging in Place in Subsidized Housing* (1993); *Changes in Extended Care in U.S. Public Housing,* and *Assisted Living in Public Housing: A Case Study of Mixing Frail Elderly and Younger Persons with Chronic Mental Illness and Substance Abuse Histories* (1998).

Robert Jenkens, Vice President at NCB Development Corporation (NCBDC), provides policy and development consulting to states, communities, and organizations interested in promoting affordable assisted living. Jenkens and NCBDC provide these services through the Robert Wood Johnson funded Coming Home Program. The Coming Home Program concentrates on key policy areas and development issues impacting the availability and quality of affordable assisted living, including state regulations and monitoring programs, state reimbursement policies, state housing finance agency programs, and related federal programs. Prior to joining NCBDC, Jenkens was the Real Estate Development Manager for Assisted Living Concepts, Inc. (ALC), overseeing the development of assisted living projects serving moderate income and Medicaid eligible tenants. Before joining ALC, Jenkens was a senior analyst at the AARP's Public Policy Institute, focusing on assisted living and livable community policy issues, model standards, and quality initiatives.

Jenkens received his Bachelor of Architecture from Cornell University's College of Architecture, Art and Planning, with an emphasis on residential care for older persons. He received a Master of Science in Real Estate Development from Massachusetts Institute of Technology, with an emphasis on developing affordable assisted living. He also studied public policy at Harvard University's John F. Kennedy School of Government.

Andrew Kochera is a Senior Policy Advisor with the Independent Living/Long Term Care Team of the Public Policy Institute at AARP. His areas of research include housing policy, consumer preferences, and demographics. He is also one of AARP's principle staff persons for issues related to Home Modification, Universal Design, Smart Growth and Livable Communities. His recent AARP publications include: "Accessibility and Visitability Features in Single-Family Homes: A Review of State and Local Activity" and "Serving the Affordable Housing Needs of Older Low-Income Renters:

A Survey of Low-Income Housing Tax Credit Properties." He was a contributor to AARP's "Beyond 50.03: A Report to the Nation on Independent Living and Disability." He is also the staff project leader for the upcoming revision to AARP's "Livable Communities: An Evaluation Guide."

Prior to AARP, Mr. Kochera served as the Director of Survey Analysis at the National Association of Home Builders. While there he published several articles on demographics and remodeling activity and was one of the principle staff for "What Today's Home Buyers Want." He was also responsible for surveys on market activity and housing affordability. Kochera has a BA from Trinity University and an MA in Economics from the University of Maryland, College Park.

Phoebe S. Liebig, PhD, is Associate Professor of Gerontology and Public Administration at the University of Southern California. Dr. Liebig's research interests are focused on state-policy issues related to assistive technology and home modifications, housing and long-term care for older adults and persons with disability, tax policy and the elderly, state-local relations in aging and disability services, and the roles of aging interest groups in the policy process. In addition, she has conducted research on aging issues and programs in India, an outcome of her Fulbright Senior Scholar award in 1997-1998.

She is co-editor, with S. I. Rajan, of *An Aging India: Perspectives, Prospects and Policies* (Haworth Press, 2003); with Jon Pynoos of *Housing Frail Elders: International Policies, Perspectives and Prospects* (John Hopkins Press, 1995); and with William Lammers of *California Policy Choices for Long-Term Care* (Andrus Gerontology Center, University of Southern California, 1990).

She has made more than 200 presentations at scientific and professional meetings and is the author of numerous book chapters, encyclopedia articles and journal articles. She has published in *Journal of Aging & Social Policy, Journal of Housing for the Elderly, Technology and Disability, Journal of Applied Gerontology, The Gerontologist,* and *Indian Journal of Social Development.*

Her professional experience includes Senior Policy Analyst, Economic Team, Public Policy Institute, AARP; Director of the Pacific Geriatric Education Center at the USC School of Medicine; Planning Director and Policy Analyst at the Andrus Gerontology Center; and Staff (Summer) to the U.S. Congress, House of Representatives Select Committee on Aging. She is the recipient of the 2003 Clark Tibbitts Award for leadership in the field of aging and is a Fellow of both the Gerontological Society of America and the Association for Gerontology in Higher Education.

Lindsay M. Maher is a project manager for NCB Development Corporation (NCBDC) where she manages grants, marketing, and communications efforts for NCBDC's Community Solutions Group (CSG). CSG is the technical assistance arm of NCBDC that provides policy and development consulting to states, communities, and organizations interested in promoting affordable housing with services for low-income, frail seniors and individuals with disabilities. She recently published "Coming Home: Creating Affordable Assisted Living for Low-Income Seniors" in *Social Policy Magazine* (Winter 2000, with David Nolan).

Christy M. Nishita, PhD, is a postdoctoral researcher at the University of Southern California's Andrus Gerontology Center. She received her PhD in Gerontology from the Leonard Davis School of Gerontology at USC. Her research interests include supportive housing, long-term care service delivery, and self-care. Her most recent publications include "Housing and the Continuum of Care" in Evashwick's *The Long-Term Continuum of Care* and "The Cost and Financing of Home Modifications in the United States" in the *Journal of Disability Policy Studies* (2003, with Jon Pynoos).

Claudia E. Oakes, MS, OTR/L, is a doctoral candidate with a concentration in Gerontology at the University of Connecticut in the School of Family Studies. She is an occupational therapist with 16 years experience in a variety of health care settings. Her research interests include home safety for the elderly and autonomy in senior housing. She completed her Master's degree at the University of Connecticut in the School of Allied Health and joined the faculty of the Occupational Therapy Department at the University of Hartford. Ms. Oakes is a member of the American Occupational Therapy Association and the Gerontological Society of America. She has presented at national conferences of both groups and has published in *The Gerontologist.*

Janet O'Keeffe, DrPH, RN, has over 15 years experience as a researcher and policy analyst on a wide range of aging, disability, long-term care, and health policy issues. She is a nationally recognized expert on long-term care policy and the Medicaid program.

Before coming to RTI, Dr. O'Keeffe was a Senior Social Scientist in the Office of the Assistant Secretary for Planning and Evaluation's (ASPE's) Division on Disability, Aging, and Long-Term Care. While there, she developed a *Primer on Medicaid Home and Community Services,* which has been widely recognized as the most comprehensive source of information on the topic currently available. Prior to working at ASPE, Dr. O'Keeffe was a Senior Policy Advisor in AARP's Public Policy Institute, where she analyzed a wide range of long-term care policy issues, including methods for determining eligibility for publicly-funded long-term care services and for private long-term care insurance.

She is currently serving as the Project Director of a CMS-funded implementation evaluation of the Real Choice Systems Change Grants for Community Living Program. Systems Change Grantees are addressing a wide range of long-term care issues, including the development of affordable and accessible housing for persons with disabilities. Dr. O'Keeffe was the Project Director for two recently completed ASPE-funded projects: the first to develop a policy and research agenda to inform the development of affordable supportive housing with services; and the second to examine Medicaid's current role in providing services in residential care settings. She is currently Project Director of an ASPE-funded study on the use of negotiated risk agreements in residential care settings.

Donald L. Redfoot, PhD, has worked for the past seven years as a Senior Policy Advisor in AARP's Public Policy Institute. In this capacity, he conducts and supervises public policy research on issues related to assisted living, housing for older persons, long term care options, and reverse mortgages. Previously, Don served eight years as a lobbyist for AARP on housing and assisted living issues. He also spent a year and a half with the House of Representative's Special Committee on Aging, the Subcommittee on Housing and Consumer Interests and taught for two years with the University of Maryland's European Division.

Don has a PhD in Sociology from Rutgers University, an MA in the Social Sciences from the University of Chicago, and a BA in Sociology from Westminster College (PA). He conducted post-doctoral research at Duke University's Center for the Study of Aging and Human Development under grants from the National Institute for Mental Health and the National Institute on Aging. He has published numerous articles on aging issues in scholarly, practitioner, public policy, and popular publications.

Don resides in Billings, Montana with his wife and two children, where he continues to work as a telecommuter for AARP's Public Policy Institute.

Nancy W. Sheehan, PhD, serves as Associate Dean and Director of Graduate Studies in the School of Family Studies and directs the Center on Aging and Human Development at the University of Connecticut. Her research and writing have focused on planned residential environments for elders. She has published research addressing a wide range of housing-related issues including resident services coordination, mixed age populations in subsidized housing, and management issues in working with frail elderly residents. Her special interests involve understanding the dynamics of social environments in different types of elderly housing settings. Her most recent research examines the impact of bringing assisted living services into congregate housing on residential policies, management and staff, and residents.

Debra L. Tillery has 30 years experience in state government with a focus on health care for persons with disabilities and the elderly. She has worked with Medicaid Waivers, Older American's Act Programs, and State Aging Programs. Ms. Tillery has performed Management Surveys to assess the compliance of Area Agencies on Aging programs funded by the Older American's Act, Medicaid, and State General Revenues. She monitored new plans for Senior Center Buildings developed in cooperation with the Arkansas Development Finance Authority, and served on a review committee for the state Housing and Urban Development office to select Model Projects. Ms. Tillery has also developed and presented workshops and training for paraprofessionals on dealing with patients with hearing loss and vision loss, and completed onsite needs assessments of Medicaid Waiver applicants to develop plans of care, determine cost effectiveness of services, and assist with provider enrollment. Ms. Tillery served as SUA Coordinator for Americans with Disabilities Act compliance, representing SUA on the Governor's Developmental Disabilities Council for ten years.

Joshua M. Wiener, PhD, is a Fellow and Program Director for Aging, Disability and Long-Term Care at RTI International. He is the author or editor of eight books and over 100 articles on health care for older people, long-term care, Medicaid, health reform, health care rationing, and maternal and child health. Prior to coming to RTI International, Dr. Wiener did policy analysis and research for the Urban Institute, the Brookings Institution, the Health Care Financing Administration, the Massachusetts Department of Public Health, the Congressional Budget Office, the New York State Moreland Act Commission on Nursing Homes and Residential Facilities, and the New York City Department of Health. He received his BA from the University of Chicago and his PhD from Harvard University.

Introduction

This special volume features a set of articles focused on key issues related to the linkages between housing and supportive services for an aging U.S. population. Assuring adequate access to necessary long-term care (LTC) services is often identified as an aging issue, but the fact that housing can be a significant problem for the elderly is often overlooked by policymakers and the public at large. Even less apparent to many is the connection between the two areas, despite the fact that people's ability to receive services is often contingent on where they live. Moreover, the potential to increase the quality of both services and housing can be greatly enhanced when the two are considered together.

The subject of linking housing and supportive services is receiving more attention as states attempt to balance increasing LTC costs with the legal ramifications of the Olmstead decision.[1] In addition, consumers–both older adults and their grown children–are becoming increasingly vocal about their preferences and, like many state policymakers, are looking for examples of attractive, affordable housing-with-services options. Pressure will increase as baby boomers begin not only to help their parents make decisions but as they consider their own options as they join the ranks of older adults.

The nexus between housing and supportive services is complex; even identifying what types of services or housing are being discussed is difficult because terms mean different things to different people. This is a significant problem for policymakers concerned with funding, targeting, regulation, eval-

The Center for Home Care Policy & Research would like to thank the authors, reviewers, and meeting participants for their contributions as well as the Robert Wood Johnson Foundation for its support of this project.

[Haworth co-indexing entry note]: "Introduction." Pynoos, Jon, Penny Hollander Feldman, and Joann Ahrens. Co-published simultaneously in *Journal of Housing for the Elderly* (The Haworth Press, Inc.) Vol. 18, No. 3/4, 2004, pp. 1-4; and: *Linking Housing and Services for Older Adults: Obstacles, Options, and Opportunities* (eds: Jon Pynoos, Penny Hollander Feldman, and Joann Ahrens) The Haworth Press, Inc., 2004, pp. 1-4. Single or multiple copies of this article are available for a fee from The Haworth Document Delivery Service [1-800- HAWORTH, 9:00 a.m. - 5:00 p.m. (EST). E-mail address: docdelivery@haworthpress.com].

http://www.haworthpress.com/web/JHE
Digital Object Identifier: 10.1300/J081v18n03_01

uation, and even marketing in this area. For example, there continues to be disagreement about how "assisted living" differs from "residential care" and how both differ from "institutional care." Advances in policy and research will require clearer definitions and classifications.

In an attempt to clarify the issues related to housing and service linkages, a number of specific questions need to be addressed. What populations are being served now, what is their level of frailty, and who is being left out? What types of services are needed by whom? What services might be needed in the future? What are the sources of payment (e.g., out-of-pocket, Medicaid, other insurance)? Where are people being served? Are they living in individual or group settings? Who are the owners of the residential settings, what are their physical characteristics (e.g., are there private bathrooms and common spaces?), and what policies govern entrance and exit decisions? Finally, exactly what types of services are being provided, who is providing them, and how are they packaged? Are services limited to "hotel services" (e.g., meals, laundry, recreation) and/or "personal assistance services" (e.g., bathing, dressing), or do they include "skilled care" (e.g., service coordination, medication management, 24-hour nurse oversight)? In addressing these questions, the articles in this volume analyze the issues, identify barriers to progress, and generate specific recommendations on ways to better link housing and supportive services for older adults.

The seven articles in this collection are an outgrowth of a national conference on housing and supportive services sponsored by the Center for Home Care Policy & Research of the Visiting Nurse Service of New York. The conference, entitled "Linking Housing and Long-Term Care Services for Older Adults," was funded by the Robert Wood Johnson Foundation and held in New York City over a 2-day period in February 2004.

In "Homes of Choice: Towards More Effective Linkages Between Housing and Services," Jon Pynoos, Phoebe Liebig, Dawn Alley, and Christy M. Nishita present the argument for increased development of supportive housing for older adults, while examining the barriers that states face in moving that development forward. The authors propose a range of strategies that states should consider pursuing and recommend areas for future research in the growing area of supportive housing. Among their many recommendations, they suggest the most effective strategies for states are to increase service coordination in multi-unit housing, to retrofit existing buildings and modify existing units, and to use Medicaid waivers in conjunction with SSI and Section 8 vouchers to make assisted living affordable in both existing and new developments.

In "Public Funding for Long-Term Care Services for Older People in Residential Care Settings," Janet O'Keeffe and Joshua Wiener focus on the issues related to providing a variety of housing and service options to the Medicaid population. They address topics ranging from current Medicaid reimbursement rates and regulations to the ability of residential care facilities to provide quality care and support aging in place. In their analysis they examine a number of difficult policy trade-offs and observe that states need to find the appropriate balance between competing goals, which will vary depending on their fiscal and political environments as well as the unique characteristics of their current LTC systems.

Two case studies included in this volume–"Public Policy Initiatives Addressing Supportive Housing: The Experience of Connecticut" by Nancy Sheehan and Claudia Oakes and "Supportive Housing Initiatives in Arkansas" by Debra Tillery–illustrate how policies aimed at linking housing and services play themselves out at the state and local levels. These case studies provide a wealth of information about specific initiatives that have been successful in two very different geographical and political contexts. Notably, a common theme in both case studies is that strong leadership and the ability to develop key partnerships were at least as important as identifying and creatively using various funding sources.

Donald Redfoot and Andrew Kochera's "Targeting Services to Those Most at Risk: Characteristics of Residents in Federally Subsidized Housing" focuses on the interrelationship of factors associated with nursing home admission, the availability of subsidized housing and Medicaid eligibility. The article makes a strong case that because of its unique population, subsidized housing should play an integral role in LTC reform.

The importance of the environmental perspective is emphasized in Leonard Heumann's "Assisted Living for Lower-Income and Frail Older Persons from the Housing and Built Environment Perspective." Heumann argues that the next wave of care management needs to be holistic and include environmental care assessment, repair and renovation management in addition to the more traditional medical and social services management services found in current LTC settings.

The final article provides a detailed look at how to create affordable assisted living facilities for older persons eligible for Medicaid services. Robert Jenkens, Paula Carder and Lindsay Maher's "The Coming Home Program: Creating a State Road Map for Affordable Assisted Living Policy, Programs, and Demonstrations" describes the successful components of the national Coming Home Program as well as four case studies that emphasize different finance and regulatory approaches to provide lessons learned for developers, state agencies, and advocates of affordable assisted living.

This special publication can help state, federal, and local policymakers pursue projects that strengthen linkages between housing and supportive services. The experience of the highlighted programs underscores the importance of partnering, the necessity of crossing administrative boundaries, and the pay-off of innovation in the cause of better meeting the needs of frail older persons. The authors urge us to learn from both past mistakes and successes in order to overcome barriers and to pursue strategies that will allow us to replicate what has been done well–on larger scales, when possible. Their recommendations include building public/private partnerships, ensuring consumers have a voice, improving communication between housing and service agencies, being creative with funding sources, finding a regulatory framework that can monitor quality while preserving consumer choice, and continuing to invest in vital policy-related research. Following such recommendations can help provide more optimal residential choices for the increasing number of frail older adults.

Jon Pynoos, PhD
Penny Hollander Feldman, PhD
Joann Ahrens, MPA
Editors

NOTE

1. The Supreme Court's 1999 *Olmstead v. L. C.* decision requires states to provide services "in the most integrated setting appropriate to the needs of qualified individuals with disabilities." <http://www.cms.hhs.gov/olmstead/default.asp>

Homes of Choice:
Towards More Effective Linkages
Between Housing and Services

Jon Pynoos
Phoebe Liebig
Dawn Alley
Christy M. Nishita

SUMMARY. State policymakers increasingly recognize that housing is not only an important shelter resource for older persons, but also a key element of community-based care. Over the last two decades, significant state and local activity has led to an increase in service-enriched housing for older persons. Service-enriched housing refers to living arrangements that include health and/or social services in an accessible, supportive environment. Emerging forces are leading to increased pressure

Jon Pynoos, PhD, Phoebe Liebig, PhD, Dawn Alley, BS and Christy M. Nishita, PhD, are affiliated with the National Resource Center on Supportive Housing and Home Modification, University of Southern California; and Information Brokering for Long-Term Care, a project of the Center for Home Care Policy & Research of the Visiting Nurse Service of New York.

They are grateful for the excellent research assistance of Teri Koenig and Kali Peterson, the policymakers and providers who participated in interviews for this project (see Appendix D), and the reviewers of the paper for their useful comments.

The authors would like to acknowledge the support of the Archstone Foundation and The California Endowment.

Funded by the Robert Wood Johnson Foundation.

[Haworth co-indexing entry note]: "Homes of Choice: Towards More Effective Linkages Between Housing and Services." Pynoos, Jon, Phoebe Liebig, Dawn Alley, and Christy M. Nishita. Co-published simultaneously in *Journal of Housing for the Elderly* (The Haworth Press, Inc.) Vol. 18, No. 3/4, 2004, pp. 5-49; and: *Linking Housing and Services for Older Adults: Obstacles, Options, and Opportunities* (eds: Jon Pynoos, Penny Hollander Feldman, and Joann Ahrens) The Haworth Press, Inc., 2004, pp. 5-49. Single or multiple copies of this article are available for a fee from The Haworth Document Delivery Service [1-800-HAWORTH, 9:00 a.m. - 5:00 p.m. (EST). E-mail address: docdelivery@haworthpress.com].

Digital Object Identifier: 10.1300/J081v18n03_02

for the expansion of service-enriched housing. These forces include: a growing and diverse population of older renters; older adults' preferences to age in place; the increasing frailty of subsidized housing residents; the development of assisted living (AL); the enactment of Medicaid waivers; and implementation of the Olmstead decision. Although studies have not included cost-analysis, available research demonstrates that service-enriched housing promotes resident satisfaction, successfully provides services to frail populations, and supports aging in place.

Given both limited resources and research, this article addresses how states can adequately respond to and capitalize on these forces in order to best meet the long-term needs of older adults. *[Article copies available for a fee from The Haworth Document Delivery Service: 1-800-HAWORTH. E-mail address: <docdelivery@haworthpress.com> Website: <http://www.HaworthPress.com> © 2004 by The Haworth Press, Inc. All rights reserved.]*

KEYWORDS. Long-term care, housing, aging, aging in place, public policy, assisted living, social services, supportive housing

OBJECTIVES

This paper analyzes the *potential* of service-enriched housing, as well as the *barriers* that impede its development. It identifies *strategies* to expand and improve supportive housing, including affordable AL, and analyzes *trade-offs* inherent in program planning. Finally, it discusses broader policy implications and future research.

FINDINGS

Why Should States Invest in Service-Enriched Housing?

Service-enriched housing is attractive to states because it:

- Provides alternatives to costly institutionalization.
- Helps housing sponsors create more successful tenancies by increasing resident satisfaction and decreasing resident turnover.
- Enables local service providers to deliver services more efficiently.
- Benefits residents, who can retain their independence longer in settings of their choice.
- Eases residents' transitions from one setting to another.

Research has shown that even low intensity programs involving only service coordination can support aging in place and help maintain frail older persons in residential settings. Higher intensity programs, such as AL, serve similar objectives but for people who are more severely impaired. AL programs take advantage of economies of scale associated with older persons living together, thereby potentially saving money for both states and localities.

What Barriers Slow the Development of Service-Enriched Housing?

- *Organizational barriers arise from the sheer number of agencies and entities with some responsibility for service-enriched housing.* Each operates with different incentives and resources. There is a professional divide between policy makers in health as distinct from those in housing. No one body "owns" the problem of meeting the needs of frail elders in subsidized housing, and the problem is underscored by the reality that savings that might result from health or service expenditures generally do not accrue to agencies that fund the development and operation of the housing.
- *Financing service-enriched housing is often a complex and time-consuming enterprise.* Creating service-enriched housing may require piecing together financing from numerous state, federal, and local sources such as Section 202, Low-Income Housing Tax Credits (LIHTC), Section 8 vouchers, Community Development Block Grants (CDBGs), redevelopment funds, and donated or discounted land from localities. Furthermore, senior housing competes with other funding priorities for resources. Similarly, securing funding for services adds yet another layer of complexity despite the range of possible sources available.
- *Regulations may delay housing development if the licensing and regulatory processes are uncoordinated.* States have different philosophies about the role of licensing, although in general, regulations are stricter for AL than for supportive housing. States also have varying admission and retention requirements that may or may not overlap with Medicaid waiver requirements. Perhaps the most serious regulatory impediment is related to the relationship between licensing and funding. Usually, licensure cannot be obtained until a facility is operational, but failure to obtain a state license may result in the denial of federal funds.

What Strategies Should States Follow to Improve the Availability and Affordability of Service-Enriched Housing?

States can employ a variety of strategies to overcome the barriers that impede development of service-enriched housing. Three broad organizational strategies include:

1. *Engage in strategic planning.* Strategic planning can overcome organizational barriers by:

- Incorporating service-enriched housing into state housing and LTC plans.
- Utilizing task forces to achieve specific objectives and address problems.
- Creating demonstration programs.

States have created a spectrum of service-enriched housing options for frail older persons by addressing the needs of seniors in various planning processes (e.g., consolidated plans, housing elements, aging service plans) and creating mechanisms to help implement them, such as task forces and demonstration programs.

2. *Efficiently broker resources.* States can successfully overcome financial barriers by:

- Determining how to best utilize existing resources.
- Launching an aggressive search for new funding.

States must determine how best to capitalize on available resources, including federal, state, and local funding, foundation grants, and private sources. This often means acting as a broker for local communities. States can participate in locating new funding opportunities and disseminating information on those opportunities. States can act alone or through umbrella organizations to advocate with Congress or federal agencies such as Housing and Urban Development (HUD), Department of Health and Human Services (HHS), and Administration on Aging (AoA) for new programs, increased funding, or changes in regulations. States can also provide direct technical assistance in obtaining funds.

3. *Work with housing sponsors and services providers.* States can overcome regulatory barriers by:

- Working with major provider groups to overcome regulatory barriers.
- States should regard service-enriched housing developers, both public and private, as partners, not as adversaries.
- Through offering provider incentives and creating effective partnerships among state agencies, local communities, and providers, states may be able to expand service-enriched housing more effectively.

The following more specific strategies can be used to address–either separately or in combination–the availability of supportive services, the physical environment of supportive housing, and the affordability of the housing and/or service components. Each strategy requires a different level of investment, and states must decide which strategies will best use their resources to meet specific needs.

1. *Encourage housing sponsors to include service coordinators and service linkages in existing housing by:*

   - Expanding the availability of service coordinators in HUD, Housing Finance Agencies (HFA) sponsored housing, other private housing, and naturally occurring retirement communities (NORCs).
   - Increasing services available in senior housing through stronger linkages with aging network programs.

2. *Increase the efficiency of service delivery.* States can empower providers to develop supportive housing with services that minimize duplication and encourage efficiency by:

   - Clustering services to Medicare and Medicaid home care recipients living in senior housing and NORCs.
   - Co-locating new service sites (e.g., adult day health centers and senior centers) near or even within senior housing.
   - Placing a priority on applications that incorporate services for residents as well as those that provide services to the wider community.

3. *Encourage housing sponsors to incorporate AL services into existing housing.* States can license and promote AL services for subsidized housing by:

   - Creating special mechanisms so that AL for subsidized housing is licensed as a service package.
   - Addressing the concerns of housing sponsors about the additional responsibility and effort involved in providing services.
   - Utilizing state funding to continue and expand the HUD Congregate Housing Services Program (CHSP) by providing AL services within current projects.

4. *Provide vouchers for private AL.* States can expand the range of affordable AL by:

   - Developing guidelines and mechanisms for use of vouchers in private AL.
   - Combining Medicaid waivers and Section 8 vouchers to allow very frail, low-income older persons to enter private AL facilities.

5. *Encourage health care providers to incorporate supportive housing in service programs.* States can help bridge the divide between housing and health care by:

- Providing HFA incentives to encourage service providers to develop housing near health care facilities and senior programs.
- Educating health and social service providers about the advantages of delivering services to concentrated groups of older persons in senior housing and NORCs.

6. *Retrofit housing buildings and units to make them more supportive.* States can promote accessibility and supportive features in both existing and new housing. Specific policies include:

- Working in conjunction with local code enforcement, HUD and the Department of Justice to ensure developer compliance with the Fair Housing Amendments Act (FHAA) and the Americans with Disabilities Act (ADA).
- Encouraging the use of CDBGs, HUD modernization funds, project reserve funds, and low-interest loan funds for retrofitting existing housing complexes and modifying individual units.
- Providing incentives for housing sponsors to include features based on the principles of universal design.

7. *Transform multi-unit housing into AL.* States can address regulatory issues and create mechanisms so that Medicaid waivers and other funds can be used to overcome the roadblocks that impede the conversion process by:

- Providing technical assistance to housing sponsors in assessing the financial feasibility of retrofitting, obtaining necessary commitments for Medicaid Waivers, and resolving regulatory issues.
- Using bond funds, reserves, or low-interest loans via HFAs to subsidize conversion projects.

8. *Mobilize resources to prevent affordable housing from converting to market-rate.* States and localities can work to preserve the affordable housing stock for older persons by:

- Lobbying the federal government to expand incentives for federal preservation programs.
- Providing their own incentives to current developers/owners to maintain affordable rents.
- Assisting non-profit developers to take over ownership/management of at-risk housing before it is converted to market rates.

9. *Mobilize resources to develop new supportive housing stock or establish purpose-built AL.* States can increase the supply of affordable, service-enriched housing by:

- Designating state dollars, e.g., via HFA "set asides" or housing trust funds, to build new units.
- Working with government-sponsored enterprises (e.g., Fannie Mae, Federal Home Loan Banks) to stimulate private investment, especially in rural locations.
- Providing priority in the distribution of LIHTC to projects that include service coordination, services, and universal design features.
- Streamlining funding, licensing, and regulatory processes and coordinating housing developers and service providers to promote purpose-built AL.

Policy Implications

Although this article contains many recommendations on how to proceed, experience suggests that the most effective strategies are to increase service coordination in multi-unit housing, retrofit existing buildings and modify units, and use Medicaid waivers in conjunction with SSI and Section 8 vouchers to make AL affordable in both existing and new developments.

Following are recommendations for how states should handle common "trade off" decisions around supportive housing.

- *Should states license AL as a building or as a service package?* In deciding how AL will be licensed, states must make choices that involve balancing safety with autonomy, costs with quality, and medical and social approaches. *The goal may best be achieved through licensing the facility and services together.*
- *Should states use strict eligibility criteria or more general targeting?* States can target service-enriched housing programs based on age, disability level, income, or a combination of characteristics. *Expanding eligibility criteria may allow states to provide services to a larger number of people and make service delivery more efficient.*
- *Should states build new service-enriched housing or preserve/transform existing housing?* The reality is that states probably need to do both. Older people aging in place in subsidized housing can benefit from immediate retrofitting and service linkages. On the other hand, much of the existing housing may be too expensive to retrofit and inappropriate for persons with high degrees of physical and cognitive impairments (e.g.,

Alzheimer's disease). For these segments of the population, it may be better to build new facilities such as AL or specially designed small group homes.

Consumer preferences and an aging population are creating an increasing demand for service-enriched housing, and in order to provide services effectively, states will have to expand and improve the current housing stock to make it more supportive. Expanding programs will require efficiently utilizing existing funding and developing new funding sources. Even when funding is available, however, programs are still difficult to develop without adequate state and local partnerships. Partnerships help to ensure community investment and relieve states from some of the burden of creating and managing new programs.

States should recognize that the best programs are long-term investments that require planning for future needs. Service-enriched housing programs may require new legislation, regulatory changes, and investment in housing stock. In order to reap the greatest return, these programs should be based on careful planning and needs assessments. As part of an overall approach to community-based care, service-enriched housing can provide a supportive environment that integrates shelter, health, and social services.

What Should Be the Focus of Future Research?

Future research around service-enriched housing should:

- *Focus on outcomes of different service-enriched housing options, with an emphasis on cost-effectiveness and targeting.* Specifically, research should explore who benefits most from services, how long frail older persons can be supported in different housing types, the costs of housing transitions, and the cost-effectiveness of service-enriched housing relative to institutionalization. Longitudinal research on the housing "careers" of older person as they age in place or move would be particularly useful in answering these questions.
- *Target processes that result in best practice programs.* While it is easy to find exemplary programs, it is more difficult to determine how they can be replicated. Research is needed to help states, localities, housing sponsors, and service providers anticipate issues and develop successful programs.
- *Develop the ability to measure quality in service-enriched housing.* As increasingly frail older persons age in place, it is important to balance autonomy with consumer protection by monitoring service-enriched housing quality.
- *Analyze how housing can be better aligned with the health and social services systems.*

INTRODUCTION:
HOUSING IS A LONG-TERM CARE RESOURCE

State policymakers increasingly recognize that housing is not only an important shelter resource for older persons, but also a key element of long-term care (LTC). Over the last two decades, significant state and local activity has led to an increase in service-enriched housing for older persons. For the purposes of this article, service-enriched housing refers to *living arrangements that include health and/or social services in an accessible, supportive environment.* Service-enriched housing can include group residences specifically designated for older persons, such as government-subsidized senior apartments, retirement housing and assisted living (AL). It can also include naturally occurring retirement communities (NORCs), which are made up of dwellings that were not designated for older persons but where seniors have lived for most of their adult lives ("aging in place"). NORCs can be public housing, private apartment buildings, mobile home parks, or any neighborhood with a high concentration of older persons who have aged in place.

Although the overwhelming majority of older persons in multi-unit housing live in private apartments (see Table 1), this article focuses on what can be learned from the experience of enhancing services in government-subsidized housing. Until recently, the nation's 20,000 subsidized senior housing complexes have been an underutilized resource for meeting the needs of frail older persons.

AIMS

The purpose of this article is to help policy analysts, policy makers, aging advocates, and researchers analyze:

- The potential of service-enriched housing
- Barriers that slow its development
- State strategies to:
    Overcome barriers
    Improve its availability and affordability
- Trade-offs and choices associated with these strategies
- Policy implications and future research

As states grapple with the challenges posed by a growing number of older persons, the historic gulf between housing and LTC is no longer tenable. Senior housing that is enriched with health and social services has great potential for enabling elders to age in place in their homes and communities. Despite

TABLE 1. Prevalence of Older Adults in Various Multi-Unit Housing Options

Type	# of Units or Facilities	# of Persons
Private Apartments[1]	3,011,000	3,584,000
Section 202[2]	285,000	320,000
Board and Care[3]	34,000	613,000
Assisted Living[4]	391,000	528,000

[1]For those aged 65+, Senior Commission, U.S. Census
[2]For those aged 62+, HUD User (1998) A Picture of Subsidized Households, in Bodaken & Brown
[3]Clark et al. (1994) Estimates of number of licensed board and care facilities
[4]Promatura Group (2000) for the National Investment Center for Senior Housing and Care Industry

barriers characteristic of human service delivery (e.g., fragmentation, organizational boundaries), states and localities have already demonstrated their ability to solve problems at both ends of the spectrum by expanding the supply of affordable, service-enriched housing and by implementing programs to deliver services in senior housing.

This document identifies promising state and local strategies. Its purpose is to help state policy makers, policy analysts, aging advocates, and researchers analyze the challenges and opportunities in creating service-enriched housing through the use of existing resources and generation of new ones. *Although solutions have developed over time and might be seen as unique to a given state or community's political culture, many of them are generic and, with some tailoring, can be used in a variety of states* (see Appendix A.) They are organized according to a continuum of low to high levels of investment (time, resources, and commitment) that is required of stakeholders.

The information provided is designed to enable state policymakers to better understand the issues involved in using housing as a community-based care resource, with an emphasis on improving linkages between housing and services. It focuses on the crucial roles played by state housing and aging agencies, as well as housing sponsors.

WHY SHOULD STATES INVEST IN SERVICE-ENRICHED HOUSING?

Emerging Forces Are Leading to Policy Innovation

Today, emerging forces are propelling state and local governments to promote service-enriched housing. These forces include a growing and diverse population of older renters, older adults' preferences to age in place, the increasing frailty of subsidized housing residents, the development of AL, the enactment of Medicaid waivers, and implementation of the Olmstead decision.

- The demand for a broad range of affordable service-enriched housing will continue to escalate as the older population grows. The number of senior rental households is expected to increase by 22 percent between 2000 and 2020 (Commission on Affordable Housing and Health Facility Needs for Seniors in the 21st Century, 2001). These renters represent an increasingly diverse population in terms of age, income, cultural background, and health status.
- The majority of older persons express a strong desire to remain in their own dwelling units as long as possible. This is especially true of low-income older persons and adults over age 80, whose options are very limited (AARP, 2000). Access to health and social services, coupled with environmental modifications, can increase their ability to age in place.
- The need for supportive services is growing as current residents, who have aged in place, have gradually become more frail. Nearly 25 percent of older renters have at least one functional impairment, such as difficulty preparing meals, making phone calls, paying bills, bathing, dressing, or using the bathroom (Commission, 2002). More importantly, occupants of subsidized housing report even higher rates of disability, with 40 percent of Section 202 residents reported as having at least one functional impairment (Heumann, Winter-Nelson, & Anderson, 2001).
- AL has created a residential setting that provides older people with a package of housing and services. Currently, AL primarily serves middle- and upper-income, private pay clients. However, while the average yearly fee for private AL is $32,400, 64 percent of seniors have annual incomes under $25,000 (Schuetz, 2003). In response to this gap, states are exploring AL's potential as an affordable setting for residents with high personal care needs.
- Medicaid waivers provide a mechanism for states to deliver in-home services to nursing-home eligible residents, thereby expanding the home and community-based services preferred by older consumers.
- The 1999 Supreme Court's *Olmstead v. L.C.* decision requires states to create a comprehensive working plan for placing qualified people in the most integrated settings (O'Hara & Day, 1999). States will have to expand their supply of service-enriched housing to meet its objectives.

Service-Enriched Housing Has Potential Advantages at the State and Local Levels

Almost all states have engaged in activities to develop service-enriched housing for older persons. Service-enriched housing is attractive to states because it efficiently links services with housing and provides alternatives to costly institutionalization. It also offers advantages to housing sponsors, localities, and older consumers. Providers can support viable resident communities by leveraging external resources. In particular, facilities can create connections with local governments to access existing services, including those provided by aging, social service, and health agencies. Adding services can also help create more successful tenancies by increasing resident satisfaction and decreasing resident turnover. Local service providers can take advantage of the economies of scale available in senior housing settings, thereby delivering services more efficiently. Perhaps most importantly, service-enriched housing benefits residents, who can retain their independence longer in settings of their choice. If residents must move, services can also ease their transitions to other settings.

Research Demonstrates the Benefits of Service-Enriched Housing

A small number of evaluations have been carried out over the last two decades to assess the effectiveness of different approaches to creating service-enriched housing. Although several evaluations have included an analysis of costs, none have directly addressed the issue of cost-effectiveness related to preventing or delaying institutionalization. Nevertheless, they illustrate the benefits of service-enriched housing, as well as the complexities and trade-offs involved.

Evaluations have been conducted of three types of service-enriched housing programs: the Congregate Housing Services Program (CHSP), Service Coordination (SC), and Assisted Living (AL).

Congregate Housing Service Program (CHSP): The CHSP was created in 1959 as the Department of Housing and Urban Development's (HUD) first major effort to create service-enriched housing for frail older persons living in Section 202 and public housing. CHSP sites provided services such as meals, transportation, homemaking, shopping, and service coordination. Over time, the program expanded to more than 100 sites serving approximately 6,000 residents (Golant, 2003). Funding requirements have shifted over time from sole reliance on HUD to significant cost sharing by providers and residents.

- Evaluations found that the CHSP effectively provided services to a targeted group of residents (average age 80) with significant ADL and IADL impairments.

- Participant impairment levels were similar to board and care home residents, but somewhat less than nursing home residents (Research Triangle, 1996, p. 41).
- The evaluation also indicated that outside agencies and informal caregivers provided important assistance.
- Despite the availability of services, almost half of the participants over a two-year period left the program.
- Movement to more restrictive settings was partly due to eligibility restrictions (e.g., residents' ability to feed themselves), the lack of staff to meet unscheduled needs or provide nursing care, and difficulty in supporting persons with cognitive problems.
- Although the studies did not directly focus on cost-effectiveness, the CHSP expended approximately $2,000 per capita for elderly participants and $3,900 for non-elderly disabled residents annually.
- Most participants were satisfied with the program and reported that they could not have continued to live where they were without CHSP services (Sherwood et al., 1985; Research Triangle, 1996).

In spite of these benefits, HUD has allowed CHSP five year contracts to expire in an effort to stop paying for direct services, leading one analyst to describe the program as "inactive" (Golant, 2003).

Service Coordination: In the 1980s, the Robert Wood Johnson Foundation (RWJF) created a Supportive Services Program in Senior Housing (SSPSH) demonstration project that provided incentives to state Housing Finance Agencies (HFAs) to use their excess reserves for implementing services in housing funded through HFA low-interest loans. Similar to the CHSP, service coordination was the cornerstone of SSPSH. However, SSPSH services were market-driven; residents were surveyed about their willingness to pay for their service needs. Evaluations indicated that the service coordinators successfully leveraged resources that resulted in new services for residents (Feder, Scanlon, & Howard, 1992).

Since 1993, new Section 202 housing has been required to meet residents' needs by planning for congregate services and adequate staffing, including service coordination, now an eligible operating expense. In 1999, more than 35 percent of all Section 202 facilities had a service coordinator on staff and another 40 percent reported that a service coordinator was available in the community (Heumann, Winter-Nelson, & Anderson, 2001).

Service coordinators can link with outside resources by contracting with a home care agency to provide personal care for frail residents, arranging for a case manager from the local Area Agency on Aging (AAA) to assist residents in applying for benefits, or transporting residents to senior centers, day care, and medical appointments.

Assisted Living (AL): During the late 1980s and early 1990s, AL became the most rapidly growing form of residential care for the elderly (American Seniors Housing Association, 1998). Definitions of AL vary among states because some license AL facilities, while others license AL service providers. However, most AL regulations stress two central characteristics:

1. a philosophy that emphasizes resident dignity, autonomy, and choice; and
2. the availability of services to meet scheduled and unscheduled needs 24 hours a day (Hawes, 1999).

Although AL was originally targeted at affluent elderly, by October 2002, 41 states had authorized Medicaid reimbursement for AL services and four more states were planning to approve such reimbursement (Mollica, 2002). Nevertheless, even in states that utilize Medicaid reimbursement for AL, its availability is limited and thus it is not yet a viable option for most low-income elderly.

- All of six major studies of AL had difficulty defining what falls under the rubric of AL, because it often overlaps with residential care homes, board and care, and congregate care.
- Golant (2004) points out in a meta-analysis that comparison across six studies is difficult because of methodological problems related to sampling, measurements of resident impairment, and inconsistencies in definitions, such as reasons for leaving.
- Overall, research indicates that AL residents are somewhat less physically and cognitively impaired than those in nursing homes.
- A nationally representative study found that most residents who leave AL facilities move to a higher level of care; nearly 60 percent end up in nursing homes (Phillips, Munoz, Sherman, Rose, Spector, & Hawes, 2003).

However, in Oregon's affordable AL program, with liberal skilled nursing provisions and flexible nurse delegation statutes, only 20 percent of residents move to nursing homes (Golant, 1999).

Overall, the evaluations indicate that even low intensity programs involving only service coordination can support aging in place and help maintain frail older persons in residential settings. Higher intensity programs, such as AL, serve similar objectives but for more severely impaired residents who require:

a. assistance with unscheduled activities (e.g., toileting);
b. more supervision (e.g., for dementia); and
c. more medical assistance (e.g., monitoring medications).

AL programs efficiently take advantage of economies of scale associated with older persons living together, thereby potentially saving money for both states and localities. However, AL residents are generally somewhat less physically and cognitively impaired than residents of nursing facilities. Thus the evaluations suggest the importance of utilizing a spectrum of housing options as some older people will eventually need to move to settings with more medically-oriented and intensive personal care services, even if on a short term or temporary basis. Because the evaluations did not analyze cost-effectiveness related to delaying or preventing movement to more costly nursing home settings, it is too early to determine how to target service-enriched housing effectively as an alternative to institutionalization.

WHAT BARRIERS SLOW THE DEVELOPMENT OF SERVICE-ENRICHED HOUSING?

While it is clear that states should invest in service-enriched housing, there are many barriers that need to be overcome. Housing and services have long been considered separate domains, each with its own agencies, programs, and goals. "Silos" have developed, in which each agency continues to expand its domain, without branching out to connect with other interested parties. This fragmentation is reflected in different eligibility requirements, funding mechanisms, and regulations.

Organizational Barriers Create Roadblocks

Organizational barriers arise from the sheer number of agencies and entities with some responsibility for service-enriched housing. HUD regional offices, various state-level agencies (e.g., housing, finance, community development, aging/human or social services), Public Housing Authorities (PHAs) and AAAs, and a myriad of private companies and nonprofit community organizations all have some level of involvement in financing and delivering affordable service-enriched housing. However, none is formally charged with or has the motivation or resources to assume a permanent role in coordinating or integrating a complex pool of limited resources and multiple players (Golant, 2003). Furthermore, as Newman and Anvall (1995) have observed, health and housing professionals and policy makers have different orientations, time horizons, and types of expertise. Persons with multiple perspectives are rare at any level of government. Finally, the unwillingness or reluctance of HUD and many sponsors to "own" the problem of meeting the needs of frail elders in subsidized housing is yet another barrier to developing service-enriched housing. This problem is underscored by the reality that savings that might result in health or service expenditures do not accrue to agencies that fund the development and operation of the housing.

Funding Barriers Impede Progress

Financing service-enriched housing is often a complex and time-consuming enterprise. Creating service-enriched housing may require piecing together financing from numerous state, federal, and local sources such as Section 202, Low-Income Housing Tax Credits (LIHTC), Section 8 vouchers, Community Development Block Grants (CDBGs), redevelopment funds, and donated or discounted land from localities (see Table 2). Many of these sources are susceptible to policy shifts as evidenced by 2004 administrative changes in the Section 8 voucher program, the linchpin of funding for affordable housing, that threaten to undermine its ability to assist low income persons in many markets. Furthermore, senior housing competes with other funding priorities for resources. For example, Consolidated Plans and Housing Elements that state and local governments use to identify priorities often do not identify service-enriched housing as a need.

Similarly, securing funding for services adds yet another layer of complexity despite the range of possible sources available (see Table 3). For example, Older Americans Act funds and Social Service Block Grants are two flexible sources allocated at the local level that can be used for a wide range of purposes (e.g., meals, health screening, and transportation). Housing developers and managers can create relationships with local service agencies so residents have access to these services. Sponsors that develop service-enriched housing, however, are often concerned that such funding may be unreliable and that service agencies cannot make long-range commitments. Although Medicaid primarily pays for nursing home care, it can also be used to fund health-related services in service-enriched housing, such as health screening, home health, durable medical equipment, and physician visits. Medicaid waivers are used to fund a variety of home and community-based services, including environmental modification, transportation, and personal care. Services provided under waivers can be very flexible depending on the Medicaid optional services a state chooses to cover.

However, waiver eligibility is restricted because beneficiaries must meet means-tested income and asset requirements, as well as state requirements for nursing home entrance, usually based on functional impairments. Moreover, waivers are limited to a specified number of participants and often geographically restricted.

TABLE 2. Housing Funding Sources for Service-Enriched Housing

Name of Program	Description	Eligibility
Affordable Housing Trust Funds	Established by legislation, ordinance or resolution to receive public or private revenues that can only be spent on affordable housing.	State and locally-determined
Community Development Block Grant Program	Provides HUD funds to states and localities to further community and economic development.	State and locally-determined
Home Investment Partnership Program	Provides HUD funds to states and localities to meet strategic goals defined by Consolidated Plan on a needs-based formula.	State and locally-determined
HUD Section 202 Program for Non-Profit Housing Sponsors	Provides rental units and may include supportive services such as meals, transportation, and service coordination.	Very low-income persons age 62 or older
Low-Income Housing Tax Credit Program	Provides tax credits to developers who invest in affordable housing; currently the largest funding source for affordable housing.	State-determined
Mortgage Revenue Bonds and 501(C)(3) Tax Exempt Bonds	Provides bonds for developers through state HFA.	State-determined
Public and Subsidized Housing	Refers to rental units financed by HUD. Families or individuals pay no more than 30 percent of their income on rent.	Low-income families or individuals of all ages
Section 8 Certificates/Vouchers	Covers the difference in rent above 30 percent of the income of the family/individual to live in HUD approved private or subsidized housing.	Low-income families or individuals of all ages

Regulatory Barriers Delay Development

Regulations may delay housing development if the licensing and regulatory processes are uncoordinated. In general, regulations are stricter for AL than for supportive housing. For example, the HUD Assisted Living Conversion Program (ALCP) illustrates the problems related to resolving regulations across agencies and levels of government. In 2000, HUD created this program to provide grants to Section 202 properties for physical conversion into AL facilities. In particular, ALCP funds are allocated for physical retrofitting to meet federal accessibility and state licensure standards, but they cannot be used to fund AL services. *Securing service funding represents a significant challenge for housing sponsors, who must demonstrate commitments from other sources to cover service costs.*

TABLE 3. Service Funding Sources for Service-Enriched Housing

Name of Program	Description	Eligibility
Medicaid	Funds health care services including health screening, medication management, transportation, some personal care, nursing home care.	Means-tested low-income individuals of all ages
Medicaid Waivers	Funds non-institutional LTC services including health-related expenses, food preparation, personal care, housekeeping, transportation.	Means-tested low-income individuals who meet state nursing home eligibility criteria
Medicare	Funds health care services including post-acute home care, skilled therapy services, medical social services, durable medical equipment.	Age 65 or over
Older Americans Act	Provides services through the Area Agency on Aging including meals, transportation, health screening, case management, other services.	Age 60 and over targeted to persons with greatest social & economic disadvantage
Service Coordination	Provides HUD service coordinators in Section 202 and public housing buildings with sufficient percentage of frail residents.	HUD senior housing residents
Social Services Block Grants	Provides HHS funds to states to promote self-sufficiency, delay institutionalization for all ages.	State-determined

Furthermore, ALCP projects are required to obtain AL licensure upon completion. Although this licensure requirement is intended to ensure quality among grant recipients, it leads to a variety of complications. First, AL licensure varies widely by state. State regulations may define AL based on service provision, facility characteristics, or level of care (Mollica & Jenkens, 2001). Only about half of states use the term "assisted living"; the rest refer to "residential care facilities," "boarding homes," etc. (American Seniors Housing Association, 2002). States also *have varying admission and retention requirements that may or may not overlap with Medicaid waiver requirements.*

Additionally, states have different philosophies about the role of licensing. In Michigan, for example, licensure has been promoted by the private sector for marketing purposes, with less emphasis on quality control measure (J. Maguire, personal communication, August 2, 2003). In other states, licensing is a key mechanism for ensuring quality of care. These complexities have resulted in sponsors in some states experiencing difficulties in satisfying ALCP licensing requirements. Perhaps the *most serious regulatory impediment is related to the relationship between licensing and funding. Usually, licensure cannot be obtained until the facility is operational, but failure to obtain the state license results in the loss of HUD funds* (Schuetz, 2003).

Sponsors using ALCP funds have succeeded in expanding the supply of affordable AL, but they have had to work through a number of regulatory barriers in the process, which may have contributed to unexpectedly high costs (Van Ryzin, 2002). The ALCP is just one example of the importance of coordinating regulations across agencies at the state, federal, and local levels to avoid delays. At the local level, zoning and NIMBY ("Not in My Back Yard") attitudes may further complicate development.

RECOMMENDED STATE STRATEGIES

States can employ a variety of strategies to overcome the barriers that impede development of service-enriched housing. First we discuss three broad organizational strategies: planning, brokering and partnering. Then we discuss nine specific strategies that address separately or in combination the physical environment of supportive housing, the availability of supportive services and the affordability of the housing and/or service components.

Organizational Strategies

1. *Engage in strategic planning*

Strategic planning can overcome organizational barriers by:

- Incorporating service-enriched housing into state housing and LTC plans.
- Utilizing task forces to achieve specific objectives and address problems.
- Creating demonstration programs.

States such as New York and Massachusetts have been able to build on senior housing as a platform for services because they have spent decades developing and maintaining an affordable housing stock (see the case study on New York in Appendix B). These states have created a spectrum of service-enriched housing options for frail older persons by addressing the needs of seniors in various planning processes (e.g., consolidated plans, housing elements, aging service plans) and creating mechanisms to help implement them, such as task forces and demonstration programs.

Initiatives in Iowa, Massachusetts, and Michigan, for example, emerged from state task forces created to address service-enriched housing. One strategy in implementing task forces is to require all HFA grantees or Older Americans

Act (OAA) service providers to teleconference on a regular basis, perhaps even monthly, to solve problems and share information. States have used demonstration programs as a mechanism to plan, develop and test new approaches. For example, Florida has experimented with financing techniques to determine how to distribute Medicaid funds most efficiently. Michigan's AL waiver program grew out of a demonstration program originally serving 20 residents.

2. *Efficiently broker resources*

States can successfully overcome financial barriers by:

• Determining how to best utilize existing resources.
• Launching an aggressive search for new funding.

States must determine how best to capitalize on available resources, including federal, state, and local funding, foundation grants, and private sources. This often means acting as a broker for local communities. In some cases, states play a very direct role in brokering resources by providing technical assistance. For instance, if a locality in Montana donates land for service-enriched housing development, the state works directly with a private corporation to arrange development. In Iowa, the state HFA works with housing developers to secure funding for both housing and services.

States can also participate in locating new funding opportunities. States that disseminate information on federal funding opportunities may help secure this funding for communities. Additionally, states can act alone or through umbrella organizations (e.g., Council of State Housing Agencies, National Association of State Units on Aging, National Governors Association) to advocate with Congress or federal agencies such as HUD, HHS, and AoA for new programs, increased funding, or changes in regulations. States can also be instrumental in garnering foundation resources. The RWJF SSPSH and Coming Home programs have helped many states to expand service-enriched housing options for the elderly.

At a program-design level, states can consider how best to distribute available resources through targeting and funding mechanisms. For instance, providing services at a range of prices based on income level, rather than only for the very poor, may provide the necessary economies of scale to deliver services in rural settings. In Minnesota, public and private buildings in which at least 80 percent of residents are over age 55 must register with the Department of Health. Residents of all income levels then receive county-sponsored case management to assist them in locating services.

3. *Work with housing sponsors and service providers*

States can overcome regulatory barriers by working with major provider groups. States should regard service-enriched housing developers, both public and private, as partners, not as adversaries. Regulatory battles over AL are a case in point. States should consider the impact of regulations on service-enriched housing development. Many of the cost-saving solutions described in this article, such as service clustering and co-location, require sponsor involvement and investment. Through offering provider incentives and creating effective partnerships among state agencies, local communities, and providers, states may be able to expand service-enriched housing more effectively.

Specific State Strategies to Improve the Availability and Affordability of Service-Enriched Housing

States use a variety of strategies to create service-enriched housing. Each strategy requires a different level of investment, and states must decide which strategies will best use their resources to meet specific needs. While some states have done very little to develop such options, others have created a substantial range. Clearly, when it comes to the development and expansion of service-enriched housing, one size does not fit all (see Appendix C). We discuss nine main strategies according to level of investment (see Table 4).

1. Encourage housing sponsors to *include service coordinators* and *service linkages* in existing housing

TABLE 4. The Continuum of State Strategies for Service-Enriched Housing

1. Encourage housing sponsors to include service coordinators and service linkages in existing housing.	*Lower level of investment*
2. Increase the efficiency of service delivery.	
3. Encourage housing sponsors to incorporate AL services into existing housing.	
4. Provide vouchers for private AL.	
5. Encourage health care providers to incorporate supportive housing into service programs.	
6. Retrofit housing buildings and units to make them more supportive.	
7. Transform multi-unit housing into AL.	
8. Mobilize resources to prevent affordable housing from converting to market prices.	
9. Mobilize resources to develop new supportive housing stock or establish purpose-built AL.	*Higher level of investment*

- Expand the availability of service coordinators in subsidized (e.g., HUD, HFA) and other privately sponsored housing.
- Increase services available in senior housing through stronger linkages with aging network programs.

As discussed earlier, service coordination is an effective strategy to assess resident needs and link services to housing. Service coordination is primarily available in HUD-financed Section 202 and public housing. However, as the original RWJ Supportive Services in Senior Housing demonstration found, service coordination can also benefit residents of other types of projects, including those financed by HFAs. Currently, only 15 percent of housing financed under the Low Income Tax Credit Program includes service coordination, indicating the potential for expansion (Kochera, 2002). HFAs should find ways to allow and encourage sponsors of senior housing to include service coordination as an allowable operating expense, use reserves in order to pay for it, or find other mechanisms to make it available. Conversely, State Units on Aging can encourage Area Agencies on Aging to provide service coordinators to existing housing or assign case managers to complexes with large numbers of older residents to perform a similar function.

2. Increase the *efficiency* of service delivery

States can empower providers to develop supportive housing with services that minimize duplication and encourage efficiency by:

- Clustering services to Medicare and Medicaid home care recipients living in senior housing and NORCs.
- Co-locating new service sites (e.g., adult day health centers and senior centers) near or even within senior housing.
- Placing a priority on applications for new housing that incorporate services for residents as well as those that provide services to the wider community.

Clustering services takes advantages of economies of scale by consolidating fragmented services for multiple clients. This strategy can reduce travel time and costs, allowing for more efficient service delivery. For example, the New York City Human Resources Administration changed its traditional provision of personal care services to groups of subsidized-housing residents by reducing the number of home attendant agencies serving any one building. The attendants were assigned to a cluster of residents in a building, thereby saving time by letting workers move from one resident to another nearby instead of spending long blocks of time with each individual. This program saved money, although those residents with high impairment may have received less uninterrupted care (Feldman, Latimer, & Davidson, 1996). Clustering services can be facilitated by placing residents with high service needs in one wing or floor of a facility.

Clustering services can also take place on a neighborhood basis. For example, naturally occurring retirement communities (NORCs), consisting of neighborhoods with high concentrations of older people are ideal places to add service coordinators and other personnel. These communities often have as their basis apartment buildings not initially planned for older persons but in which residents have aged in place. They also include areas from which younger people have migrated out and ones in which older people have in-migrated. Currently, AoA along with the RWJ Foundation has a demonstration project to add services to NORCs.

Co-locating services, by providing multiple services at the same site, pools resources and saves money. States can encourage co-location by coordinating state programs with housing sites. For instance, several Section 202 housing sites in Illinois also include an OAA-funded state Case Coordination Unit, providing case management services to older residents in the buildings as well as in the broader community. State Units on Aging can recommend that programs such as nutrition sites and day care be located within or adjacent to senior housing as a way to make them readily available to residents, taking advantage of resident volunteers and reducing expenses associated with transporting residents to such programs. At the same time, HFAs can provide incentives for housing sponsors to locate senior housing near services and shopping. Alternatively, space can be included for such programs and services on-site as well as commercial stores (e.g., groceries, dry cleaning, and restaurants) on the first floor of buildings, a common approach used for elderly service housing in Scandinavian countries (see the case study on Washington in Appendix B.)

3. Encourage housing sponsors to *incorporate AL services* into existing housing

States can find ways to license and promote AL services for subsidized housing:

- Create special mechanisms so that AL for subsidized housing is licensed as a service package.
- Address the concerns of housing sponsors about the additional responsibility and effort involved in providing services.

- Utilize state funding to continue and expand the HUD CHSP by providing AL services within current projects.

States such as New York and Connecticut license AL service providers and have developed programs in which housing residents enrolled in the expiring Congregate Housing Services Program (CHSP), along with other residents who are eligible for nursing home admission can receive AL services (see Sheehan and Oakes, this volume).

4. Provide vouchers for private AL

In order to expand the range of affordable AL, states can develop guidelines and mechanisms for use of vouchers in private AL. Michigan has developed a demonstration program, combining Medicaid waivers and Section 8 vouchers, to allow very frail, low-income older persons to enter private AL facilities. The Department of Community Health is responsible for the program at the state level and the Medicaid waiver agent operates the program locally (see Appendix B).

5. Encourage health care providers to *incorporate supportive housing* into their service programs

States can help bridge the divide between housing and health care by:

- Providing HFA incentives to encourage service providers to develop housing near health care facilities and senior programs.
- Educating health and social service providers about the advantages of delivering services to concentrated groups of older persons in senior housing and NORCs.

The need for strategies that link housing, health, and personal care services is paramount. Health care providers can take advantage of the economies of scale that result from incorporating senior housing into their programs. For example, some Program of All-inclusive Care for the Elderly (PACE) sites have taken steps to develop their own housing. PACE integrates Medicare and Medicaid financing to provide long-term care services that enable nursing home-eligible seniors to remain in the community.

The On Lok program, on which the PACE program was modeled, developed a Section 202 housing complex adjacent to its large day care center to serve as a residence for older persons needing more supervision and services than were available in their prior residences. Although only a few PACE sites included housing initially, many have added it nearby to more effectively meet client needs (Van Ryzin, 2002) (see the case study on Colorado in Appendix B).

6. Retrofit housing buildings and units to make them more supportive

States can promote accessibility and supportive features in both existing and new housing. Specific policies include:

- Working in conjunction with local code enforcement, HUD and the Department of Justice to ensure developer compliance with the Fair Housing Amendments Act (FHAA) and the ADA.
- Encouraging the use of CDBGs, HUD modernization funds, project reserve funds, and low-interest loan funds for retrofitting existing housing complexes and modifying individual units.
- Providing incentives for housing sponsors to include features based on the principles of universal design (UD).

Most multi-unit housing has been designed for independent older persons. Consequently, substantial physical improvements may be needed to allow older people to age in place and to facilitate service delivery. For example, entrances may need to be retrofitted for accessibility, common space provided for meals and health care services, and additional features provided in apartments to accommodate wheelchairs. In California, a state housing bond included $5 million for retrofitting existing multi-unit housing to meet the needs of disabled and frail persons. Applications for this program, many of which focused on ramps, exceeded the amount of available funds only days after it was announced, indicating the enormous latent need for these renovations.

The FHAA of 1988 and the ADA (which applies to common spaces) together require accessible entrances and common spaces, wide enough corridors for wheelchairs, accessible units, backing for grab bars in bathrooms and lowered light switches, raised electrical outlets in new multi-unit housing over four units. In housing built before the Acts were implemented, the FHAA calls for landlords to make changes in common areas for persons with disabilities, but applies the standard of "reasonable accommodation," which is vaguely defined and subject to economic constraints. The Act also allows tenants to make modifications to their individual apartments, but does not require landlords to pay for those changes.

Research has shown that home modification and assistive technology services decrease Medicaid costs and delay institutionalization (Mann et al., 1999). States and localities can help fill this gap by targeting funds from such sources as CDBG and the Older Americans Act for retrofitting buildings and adapting apartments. Medicaid waivers are also a source of environmental modifications but only about 60 percent of programs serving the elderly or disabled include them in their service package (Pynoos, Tabbarah, Angelelli, & Demier, 1998).

In making the housing stock more physically supportive, it is just as important to build new accessible and supportive housing as it is to retrofit existing housing. Even though new housing falls under the FHAA cited above, too many developers adhere only to the letter, rather than the spirit, of the law. For example, a new building may have an accessible entrance that is located in the back, far from parking, or the sidewalks may be so narrow that wheelchair use is hazardous. State and local code enforcement can prevent such problems. In cases of unresponsive developers and sponsors, states and localities can work with HUD's Fair Housing and Equal Opportunity division, to bring suits against them.

Beyond enforcing compliance with existing minimal accessibility regulations, states and localities can provide incentives for housing sponsors to follow the principles of UD. The purpose of UD is to meet the needs of all users, including older persons with functional, cognitive, and sensory impairments (e.g., vision and hearing). UD features in senior housing include walk-in showers, emergency alert systems, appropriate signage, spaces for on-site services and activities, and storage for mobility and assistive devices (e.g., wheelchairs, scooters, and walkers).

7. Transform existing multi-unit housing into AL

States can address regulatory issues and create mechanisms so that Medicaid waivers and other funds can be used to overcome the roadblocks that impede the conversion process by:

- Providing technical assistance to housing sponsors in assessing the financial feasibility of retrofitting, obtaining necessary commitments for Medicaid waivers, and resolving regulatory issues.
- Using bond funds, reserves, or low-interest loans via HFAs to subsidize conversion projects.

In states that license AL facilities, existing housing may be retrofitted to allow for service provision, using low-interest financing or HUD's AL Conversion Program (ALCP). Many subsidized housing projects already have a substantial number of residents who have limitations with ADLs and IADLs along with cognitive problems. Some projects may be prime candidates for conversion as they have efficiency units that are difficult to rent for independent seniors, but that may be suitable for frail residents, assuming that services are available, the housing is accessible, and common spaces exist for activities, meals, and service provision. States can support conversions by tailoring licensing and regulations for subsidized housing and by expediting service package development, because HUD only pays for structural retrofitting. Although there have been a number of successful conversions, many applicants for HUD's ALCP have experienced problems because of higher than expected construction costs, difficulty obtaining Medicaid waivers necessary to guarantee services or providing housing within the 30 percent income cap on Section 8 vouchers, and regulatory issues related to licensure. States can provide technical assistance to help sponsors through this maze of problems.

8. Mobilize resources to prevent affordable housing from converting to market rate prices

States and localities can work to preserve the affordable housing stock for older persons by:

- Lobbying the federal government to expand incentives for federal preservation programs.
- Providing their own incentives to current developers/owners to maintain affordable rents.
- Assisting non-profit developers to take over ownership/management of at-risk housing before it is converted to market rates.

Strategies to retain the supply of affordable housing are vital. Unfortunately, the supply is dwindling (Heumann, 2003). In many cities, public housing complexes have been torn down and replaced with smaller buildings with fewer units. In addition, federal housing contracts with private housing developers under various programs (e.g., Sections 8, 236 and 221d(3)) are expiring. After approximately 20 years, developers can opt out of the subsidized program and turn housing projects into market-rate housing, making them unaffordable for current tenants.

The federal government and some states have created programs to provide incentives to housing sponsors to stay in the program. For example, in California, the Cal HFA provides a broad range of financing tools that facilitate the acquisition, rehabilitation and preservation of federally-assisted affordable housing at risk of losing its affordability status. The California Preservation

Opportunity Program also offers short-term acquisition funds for preserving this housing.

> 9. Mobilize resources to develop new supportive housing stock and/or establish purpose-built AL

States can increase the supply of affordable, service-enriched housing by:

- Designating state dollars–e.g., via HFA "set asides" or housing trust funds–to build new units.
- Working with government-sponsored enterprises (e.g., Fannie Mae, Federal Home Loan banks) to stimulate private investment, especially in rural locations.
- Providing priority in the distribution of LIHTC to projects that include service coordination, services, and UD features.
- Streamlining funding, licensing, and regulatory processes and coordinating housing developers and service providers to promote purpose-built AL.

Strategies to increase the supply of supportive housing are essential because current production is insufficient to meet future needs. HUD has stopped financing new Section 8 senior housing, and for every Section 202 unit that became vacant in 1999, nine seniors were put on a waiting list, adding up to an 11-year wait time in larger cities (Heumann, 2003). Low-income baby boomers are a scant five years away from eligibility for senior housing. Thus, not only must states ensure retention of the current supply of affordable senior housing, but also an adequate supply of *new* senior housing for the next decade and beyond.

With the new supply of Section 202 housing reduced to approximately 6,000 units per year and other supply-side programs ended, the responsibility of increasing the annual production of government-subsidized rental units for low-income elders has shifted to state and local governments. Some states, such as Massachusetts, New York and Connecticut, historically have added to their affordable housing stock through their own state-funded programs, often via their HFAs. Many HFAs have created set asides for senior housing and state Departments of Housing and Community Development have used housing bonds to develop affordable supportive housing. States can also use federal (e.g., Federal Home Loan banks) and state funding to stimulate private investment (Golant, 2003). For example, the California Department of Housing and Community Development is authorized to use a portion of a recently passed $2.1 billion dollar housing bond issue to create affordable supportive housing. However, housing sponsors have had difficulty guaranteeing that they can provide services and currently seniors are not designated as a special needs group.

States and local governments working together and separately can stimulate the private sector to build more supportive housing. A rapidly growing method of financing housing across the nation has been the creation of state and local housing trust funds. Housing trust funds, also proposed at the federal level, are continuing and dedicated public sources of revenues, established by legislation, ordinance or resolution, which can only be spent on housing. Sources for the trusts include fees paid by developers (e.g., impact fees and in lieu fees), urban renewal funds, and foundations. Thirty-seven states have created such funds; the remaining 263 trust funds are largely run by cities and counties. They can provide zero-interest loans or gap financing for new construction as well as rehabilitation of affordable housing (Nelson, 2003).

The LIHTC is an underutilized federal resource for producing supportive housing (Golant, 2003). The LIHTC program creates affordable rental housing by offering investors a credit against federal income taxes based on the cost of acquiring, rehabilitating, or constructing low-income housing. Each state is allocated a certain amount of tax credits. These credits have been used by states such as Washington to make units affordable for 40 years, rather than the federally-required 15-year minimum. The programs are generally administered through HFAs that solicit competitive proposals based on state priorities in which points are given for specific attributes. Affordability usually requires Section 8 vouchers to subsidize tenant rents. As noted earlier, extra points in the evaluation process could be provided for projects that include service coordination, services, and UD features to increase their supportiveness and prepare for the aging in place of residents.

The efforts of several states, including Alaska, Arkansas, Florida, and Iowa (see the case studies on Alaska and Iowa in Appendix B), suggest that strategies to create purpose-built affordable AL are viable. Purpose-built AL requires significant coordination among housing developers and service providers. The Coming Home program, sponsored by the RWJF, provides grant support, technical assistance, and loans to nine states to create affordable models of rural AL linked with existing community health care systems. It is anticipated that participating states will be able to continue these efforts, similar to the long-range impact of other RWJF demonstration projects.

TRADE-OFFS AND CHOICES IN SERVICE-ENRICHED HOUSING

The previous sections highlighted state strategies to increase the service-enriched housing supply. States, localities, and older persons all benefit from these programs, but service-enriched housing is often difficult to develop. Agencies must work together to develop a range of options that serve the particular needs of older citizens in each state. However, every state has different resources and challenges. Strategies successful for a rural state may not meet the needs of a more urban state, and strategies that are successful for a state with an extensive service-enriched housing stock may not be feasible in a state with fewer resources. The following dilemmas highlight trade-offs involved in developing service-enriched housing.

1. Should States License AL as a Building or as a Service Package?

In deciding how AL will be licensed, states must make choices that involve balancing safety with autonomy, costs with quality, and medical and social approaches. Mollica (2000) has identified four regulatory models. The institutional model is based on older board and care regulations. The second, a new housing and service model, licenses facilities with apartment settings and allows varying levels of nursing care. The third, the service model, licenses services and allows existing building codes to address the housing structure. Lastly, the umbrella model involves issuing regulations that cover multiple types of housing. All of these models involve trade-offs. For example, using the service model may make it easier and less expensive for housing sponsors to incorporate services because they are not required to retrofit the physical structure. However, licensing services may result in a lack of coordination between housing and service providers, thereby not fully achieving the goal of supporting the independence and autonomy of residents. *This goal may best be achieved through licensing the facility and services together.*

2. Should States Use Strict Eligibility Criteria or More General Targeting?

States can target service-enriched housing programs based on age, disability level, income, or a combination of characteristics. For example, Medicaid waivers focus on residents who meet income and asset eligibility and functional eligibility requirements, thereby ensuring that funds are targeted to older persons most at risk of nursing home placement. Using strict eligibility criteria ensures that beneficiaries include only those who will benefit most from services, maximizing impact while limiting costs. However, such strict eligibility criteria may leave out individuals who could benefit from the program. Additionally, strict eligibility criteria may not create economies of scale necessary to provide services in rural areas or small buildings. *Expanding eligibility criteria may allow states to provide services to a larger number of people and make service delivery more efficient.*

3. Should States Build New Service-Enriched Housing or Preserve/Transform Existing Housing?

The reality is that states probably need to do both. In the short-run, a substantial amount of the subsidized housing stock is in jeopardy because of expiring federal contracts. If this situation is not ameliorated, a state can lose up to 20 percent of its affordable housing stock. Just as importantly, older people aging in place in subsidized housing can benefit from immediate retrofitting and service linkages. Many of these residents are low-income, single women who have physical and cognitive limitations. They have very few alternatives except board and care or nursing homes. On the other hand, much of the existing housing may be too expensive to retrofit and inappropriate for persons with high degrees of physical and cognitive impairments (e.g., Alzheimer's disease). For these segments of the population, it may be better to build new facilities such as AL or specially designed small group homes. Moreover, even though the first obligation is to existing tenants, preparing for the future will require developing strategic plans that analyze a range of housing and service options.

POLICY IMPLICATIONS AND FUTURE RESEARCH

In the future, service-enriched housing will become an even more important element of community-based care. States, localities, and older persons all can benefit from improved programs and policies, but, as discussed earlier, barriers impede progress. Unfortunately, little research is available to guide states about what directions to take and how best to operate service-enriched housing programs.

Policymakers Should Continue to Expand Service-Enriched Housing

First, states should recognize the great need for service-enriched housing. Consumer preferences and an aging population are creating an increasing demand, and in order to provide services effectively, states will have to expand and improve the current housing stock to make it more supportive. Although this report contains many recommendations on how to proceed, *experience suggests that the most effective strategies* are to increase *service coordination* in multi-unit housing, *retrofit* existing buildings and *modify* units, and to use *Medicaid waivers* in conjunction with SSI and Section 8 vouchers to make AL affordable in both existing and new developments.

Expanding programs will require efficiently utilizing existing funding and developing new funding sources. LIHTCs represent an important source, because, in conjunction with Section 8 vouchers, they represent the largest single source of funding for affordable housing. States can use LIHTC as a tool to create new service-enriched housing by including the availability of service coordination, services and accessible features as selection criteria. Housing trust funds also hold promise, whether created at the state or local level, because they are a continuing and dedicated source of funding for affordable housing.

Even when funding is available, programs are still difficult to develop without adequate *state and local partnerships*. Partnerships help to ensure community investment and relieve states from some of the burden of creating and managing new programs.

Lastly, states should recognize that *the best programs are long-term investments that require planning for future needs*. Service-enriched housing programs may require new legislation, regulatory changes, and investment in housing stock. In order to reap the greatest return, these programs should be based on careful planning and needs assessments. As part of an overall approach to community-based care, service-enriched housing can provide a supportive environment that integrates shelter, health, and social services.

Four Research Objectives Deserve Further Consideration

Future research on service-enriched housing should:

1. *Focus on outcomes of different service-enriched housing options, with an emphasis on cost-effectiveness and targeting.* Specifically, research should explore who benefits most from services, how long frail older persons can be supported in different housing types, the costs of housing transitions, and the cost-effectiveness of service-enriched housing relative to institutionalization. Longitudinal research on the housing "careers" of older persons as they age in place or move would be particularly useful in answering these questions.
2. *Target processes that result in best practice programs.* While it is easy to find exemplary programs, it is more difficult to determine how they can be replicated. Wilden and Redfoot (2002) studied ALCP projects and found that those projects that had previously offered services encountered fewer obstacles in the conversion process. Such research can help states, localities, housing sponsors, and service providers anticipate issues and develop successful programs.
3. *Develop the ability to measure quality in service-enriched housing.* As increasingly frail older persons age in place, it is important to balance

autonomy with consumer protection by monitoring service-enriched housing quality.

4. *Analyze how housing can be better aligned with the health and social services systems.* Such an approach will be useful in overcoming the "silo" effect and promoting broader planning for the future.

REFERENCES

AARP (2000). *Fixing to Stay: A National Survey on Housing and Home Modification Issues.* Washington, DC: AARP.

American Seniors Housing Association (1998). *Seniors Housing Construction Report 1998.* Washington, DC: American Seniors Housing Association.

American Seniors Housing Association (2002). *Seniors Housing State Regulatory Handbook 2002.* Washington, DC: American Seniors Housing Association.

Branch, L.G., Coulam, R.F., & Zimmerman, Y.A. (1995). PACE evaluation: Initial findings. *Gerontologist, 35,* 349-359.

Commission on Affordable Housing and Health Facility Needs for Seniors in the 21st Century (2002). *A Quiet Crisis in America.* Washington, DC: Commission on Affordable Housing and Health Facility Needs for Seniors in the 21st Century.

Feder, J., Scanlon, W., & Howard, J. (1992). Supportive services in senior housing: Preliminary evidence on feasibility and impact. *Generations, 16,* 61-62.

Feldman, P.H., Latimer, E., & Davidson, H. (1996). Medicaid-funded home care for the frail elderly and disabled: Evaluating the cost savings and outcomes of a service delivery reform. *Health Services Research, 31,* 489-508.

Golant, S.M. (1999). The promise of assisted living as a shelter and care alternative for frail American elders: A cautionary essay. In Schwarz, B. (Ed.) *Aging, Autonomy, and Architecture: Advances in Assisted Living* (pp. 32-59) Baltimore, MD: Johns Hopkins University Press.

Golant, S.M. (2003). Political and organizational barriers to satisfying low-income U.S. seniors' need for affordable rental housing with supportive services. *Journal of Aging & Social Policy, 15,* 4, 21-48.

Golant, S.M. (2004). Do impaired older persons with health care needs occupy U.S. assisted living facilities? An analysis of six national studies. *Journal of Gerontology, Social Sciences, 50B*(2), S68-S79.

Hansen, J.C. (1999). Practical lessons for delivering integrated services in a changing environment: The PACE model. *Generations, 23,* 22-28.

Hawes, C. (1999). A key piece of the integration puzzle: Managing the chronic care needs of the frail elderly in residential care settings. *Generations, 23,* 489-508.

Heumann, L. (2003). *Comments: Aging in Place Reconsidered.* Prepared for the Gerontological Society of America Annual Meeting, November 2003.

Heumann, L., Winter-Nelson, K., & Anderson, J. (2001). *The 1999 National Housing Survey of Section 202 Elderly Housing.* Washington, DC: AARP.

Kochera, A. (2002). *Serving the Affordable Housing Needs of Older Low-Income Renters: A Survey of Low-Income Housing Tax Credit Properties.* Washington, DC: AARP.

KRA Corporation (1996). *Evaluation of the Service Coordinator Program.* Washington, DC: U.S. Department of Housing and Urban Development.

Mann, W., Ottenbacher, K., Fraas, L., Tomita, M., & Granger, C. (1999). Effectiveness of assistive technology and environmental interventions in maintaining independence and reducing home care costs for the frail elderly. *Archives of Family Medicine, 8,* 210-217.

Mollica, R.L. (2002). *State Assisted Living Policy 2002.* Princeton, NJ: Robert Wood Johnson Foundation.

Mollica, R.L. & Jenkens, R. (2001). *State Assisted Living Practices and Options: A Guide for State Policy Makers.* Princeton, NJ: Robert Wood Johnson Foundation.

Mollica, R.L. (2000). *State Assisted Living Policy: 2000.* Portland, ME: National Academy for State Health Policy.

Nelson, A.C. (2003). Top ten state and local strategies to increase affordable housing supply. *Housing Facts and Findings, 5,* 1, 4-7.

Newcomer, R., Harrington, C., & Kane, R. (2002). Challenges and accomplishments of the second-generation Social Health Maintenance Organization. *Gerontologist, 42,* 543-852.

Newman, S.J., & Envall, K. (1995) *Effects of Supports on Sustaining Older Disabled Persons in the Community.* Washington, DC: AARP.

O'Hara, A., & Day, S. (2001). *Olmstead and Supportive Housing: A Vision for the Future.* Washington, DC: Center for Health Care Strategies, Inc.

Phillips, C.D., Munoz, Y., Sherman, M., Rose, M., Spector, W., & Hawes, C. (2003). Effects of facility characteristics on departures from assisted living: Results from a national study. *Gerontologist, 43,* 690-696.

Pynoos, J. (1998). *Increasing Housing Options for Frail Older Persons: State Roles and Strategies.* San Francisco, CA: American Society on Aging.

Pynoos, J. (1992). Linking federally assisted housing with services for frail older persons. *Journal of Aging & Social Policy, 4,* 157-177.

Pynoos, J. & Golant, S. (1996). Housing and living arrangements for the elderly. In Binstock, R. & George, L. (Eds.). *Handbook of Aging and the Social Sciences.* (4th ed.) (pp. 303-324). San Diego, CA: Academic Press.

Pynoos, J., Tabbarah, M., Angelelli, J., & Demier, M. (1998). Improving the delivery of home modifications. *Technology and Aging, 8,* 3-14.

Research Triangle (1996). *Evaluation of the New Congregate Housing Services Program: Second Interim Report.* Research Triangle Park, NC.

Schuetz, J. (2003). *Affordable Assisted Living: Surveying the Possibilities.* Cambridge, MA: Joint Center for Housing Studies at Harvard University.

Sheehan, N. (1999). The Resident Services Coordinator Program: Bringing Service Coordination to Federally Assisted Senior Housing. *Journal of Housing for the Elderly, 13,* 35-49.

Sheehan, N. & Oakes, C.E. (2003). Bringing assisted living services into congregate housing: Residents' perspectives. *Gerontologist, 43,* 766-770.

Sherwood, S., Morris, J.N., Sherwood, C.C., Morris, S., & Bernstein, E. (1985). *Final Report of the Evaluation of Congregate Housing Services Program.* Boston, MA: Hebrew Rehabilitation Center for the Aged.

Smith, L.A. & Pynoos, J. (2002). More than shelter: Benefits and concerns for people in HIV/AIDS housing. *Journal of HIV/AIDS & Social Services, 1*(1), 63-80.

Van Ryzin, J. (2002, Summer). From independent to assisted living: Not-for-profit senior communities blaze a trail in AL conversions. *Best Practices*, 24-28.

Wilden, R. & Redfoot, D. (2002). *Adding Assistive Living Services to Subsidized Housing: Serving Frail Older Persons with Low Incomes.* Washington, DC: AARP.

APPENDIX A
Housing and Services: State Program Examples

State	Name of Program	Housing Setting	Services Provided	Eligibility	Funding
AK	Rural Assisted Living Program	Purpose-Built Assisted Living Facility	Assisted living services provided by the Tribal Health Entity	Medicaid, Medicaid waiver	*Housing:* Section 202, Section 8, SSI, RWJF Coming Home grant, consumer fees/rent, LIHTC, HOME, State funding, CDBG, USDA-rural development, Federal Home Loan Bank, Section 232 *Services:* Medicaid, Medicaid waivers, OAA, Social Service Block Grants, Private pay
AR	Coming Home Assisted Living	Section 202	Assisted living services	Medicaid waiver, nursing home eligible	*Housing:* RWJF Coming Home grant, HOME, LIHTC, Home Loan Bank, HUD 202, Consumer fees/rent, Section 8 *Services:* Private pay, Medicaid, and Medicaid waiver
CT	Resident Service Coordinator	Section 202	Service coordination	All affordable housing residents	*Housing:* HUD 202 *Services:* HUD Service Coordination
CT	Assisted Living in Congregate Housing	State funded congregate housing	Assisted living services	Medicaid waiver, NH eligible	*Housing:* State funding *Services:* Medicaid waiver, OAA, state subsidies
IA	Affordable Assisted Living Program	HUD Section 202 conversions	Assisted living services	Subsidized housing residents to meet Medicaid requirements.	*Housing:* RWJF Coming Home Grant, USDA - rural development, LIHTC, HOME, HUD, State Senior Living Program grants *Services:* OAA, Food Stamps, Medicaid, Medicaid waivers, Medicare, Long-Term Care Insurance, Private pay
MA	Congregate Housing	State funded congregate housing	Meals, case management	Medicaid eligible residents	*Housing:* State funding *Services:* Medicaid, OAA
MA	Supportive Housing Program	State funded public housing	Selections from continuum of care	Medicaid eligible residents	*Housing:* Housing subsidies *Services:* OAA, Medicaid

State	Name of Program	Housing Setting	Services Provided	Eligibility	Funding
MI	Assisted Living Vouchers	Private assisted living	Assisted living services	Medicaid waiver, NH eligible residents	*Housing:* Section 8, SSI *Services:* HCBS waivers
MN	Housing with Service Registration Process (Virtual Assistance program)	Section 202, Section 8, and any apartment complex with 80% 55 years and older	Selections from continuum of care	Residents of registered structures	*Housing:* HUD 202, Section 8, SSI, Consumer fees/rent *Services:* Medicaid, Medicaid waivers, Front-End state resources for Alternative Care, Title 20, OAA, Private pay
MT	Accessible Space Inc. - Private	Private apartments	Selections from continuum of care	Medicaid eligible residents	*Housing:* Section 8, SSI, Consumer fees/rent, CDBG for structure, land donated by community *Services:* Medicaid, Medicaid waivers
NJ	Assisted Living Program in Subsidized Housing	NH, ADHC, RCF, AL, board and care, congregate, subsidized housing	Assisted living services	Medicaid waiver, NH eligible residents	*Housing:* HUD 202, SSI, Section 8, Foundations, Consumer fees/rent, LIHTC, HOME *Services:* OAA grants, Medicaid, Medicaid waivers, Private pay
NY	NY State Assisted Living Program	Congregate housing	Assisted living services	Medicaid eligible or private pay residents	*Housing:* SSI, Consumer fees/rent *Services:* Medicaid, Private pay
VT	Housing and Supportive Services (HASS) Program	State funded congregate housing	Selections from continuum of care	Residents who meet independent Living Assessment standards	*Housing:* HUD 202, Consumer fees/rent *Services:* State general fund, Medicaid, Medicaid Waivers, Private pay

APPENDIX B
Case Studies

Alaska   **Alaska Takes Care of Its Pioneers**

Pioneer Home, Fairbanks

Most of the 92 residents of the Fairbanks Pioneer Home were young children in 1913, when Alaska's State Legislature dedicated funds to create affordable housing and to provide services to any Alaskan 65 years and older. Today, the State Legislature annually provides approximately 50% of the total cost for a senior to live in an assisted living facility from its General Fund, and the senior pays the remaining costs. If there is a shortfall, the General Fund will supplement consumer payment. Through this state funding, the State of Alaska has not had to apply for HUD funding, voucher programs or Medicaid waivers to realize its commitment to every elder Alaskan.

Colorado   **What's Love Got to Do with It?**

The Retreat, Westminster

The Retreat, an assisted living (AL) community in Westminster, CO just outside of Denver, is home to 55 residents, 38 of whom are Medicaid beneficiaries. The Retreat works closely with Total Long-Term Care (TLC), a Medicaid provider that is a member of the PACE program, to provide services for Medicaid eligible residents. TLC receives $4,500 to $5,000 for each Medicaid resident from federal and state programs, and The Retreat receives the Medicaid approved rental payment of $1,600 per month. TLC provides personal care, medication supervision, health screenings that include eye and dental exams, housekeeping, assistance with ADLs, and 24 hour care for unscheduled services and emergency response.

Iowa   **Doing a Lot with a Little**

More than 50 percent of elderly Iowans cannot afford private AL.[1] With assistance from the Robert Wood Johnson Foundation Coming Home Project, Iowa addressed this problem by creating the Affordable Assisted Living Program, which is dedicated to developing AL for low to moderate-income seniors. In the Affordable Assisted Living Program, the Iowa Housing Finance Agency (HFA) provides technical assistance to potential housing developers and service providers. Technical assistance helps agencies overcome the financial and organizational obstacles in creating affordable AL. The National Cooperative Bank Development Corporation, working with the HFA, has created a revolving loan fund to off-set costs of assessment and facility pre-development. Additionally, program administrators advocate policies that support future growth of affordable AL.

Because the Iowa HFA recognized that one in four Iowans over age 75 has a monthly income of less than $884, the primary goal of the program was to create an AL option that included rent, meals, activities and medical services for less than that amount. To accomplish this goal, the Iowa HFA coordinated a task force that included HUD, USDA-Rural Development, the Departments of Human Services, Public Health, Elder Affairs, and Inspection and Appeals, as well as the AARP and several Iowan senior interest groups. The task force identified funding sources (see Table) that could be used for both the housing and service elements of AL. The Iowa HFA now assists facilities, localities and service providers in obtaining funding.

Six different demonstration sites are currently in operation or development. One unique model, Emerson Point, has built upon the Iowa Coming Home Program and created a co-located congregate meal-site. Seniors from the community are invited to socialize with residents and eat a nourishing meal twice a day, seven days a week, at a reduced cost.

Iowa's program provides an example of how states can capitalize on existing funding sources by acting as resource brokers, uniting housing developers and service providers to overcome barriers to create affordable AL.

Funding Sources for Affordable Assisted Living Program		
Rent	**Board**	**Services**
Development sources: Low Income Housing Tax Credits HUD grants, direct and guaranteed loans USDA-RD grants, direct and guaranteed loans Federal Home Loan Bank HOME funds Senior Living Program (pending legislative approval of funds) Conventional loans	*Development sources:* Grants from private foundations	*Development sources:* Senior Living Program (pending legislative approval of funds)
Operational sources: Tenant fees Section 8 USDA-RD project-based rental assistance DHS Rent Subsidy Program	*Operational sources:* Tenant fees Older Americans Act (congregate meals) Food Stamps	*Operational sources:* Tenant fees Medicaid waiver Medicaid Title XIX Medicare In-Home Health Related Care Long Term Care Insurance

Note

[1] Per Carla Pope, comparison of incomes from 2000 Census of those 75 and older to the cost of market-rate assisted living in 2001, as identified in a phone survey by Sade Owalabi, graduate student from the University of Iowa.

Michigan   Changing the Rules

Working with providers: A voucher program can only be successful if AL providers are willing to accept it. In Michigan, American House, a private AL company, was active in supporting the waiver. This led to support among other private AL providers and a willingness to accept waiver recipients. Beneficiaries can choose from a variety of both non-profit and for-profit facilities, but facilities must meet minimum services standards to qualify for the program.

Affordability: When this program began with 20 residents, affordability issues quickly surfaced. Although the Medicaid waiver covered AL services, facilities were not able to provide room and board under the Section 8 voucher income cap. In response, state aging and housing officials successfully influenced Congress to remove the cap, allowing recipients to contribute more money to cover room and board costs. Administrators report this change was crucial to the program's success (S. Kritzman, personal communication, June 9, 2003).

Demand: Demand can quickly outstrip program capacity, particularly when using Medicaid waivers. The program now serves 60 residents in three counties, with a waiting list of 275 applicants. Although administrators would like to expand the program, the number of waivers available limits expansion.

New York   Services Across the Board

With one of the most expensive U.S. housing markets and a population clustered in dense urban settings, New York has a significant number of elderly people aging in place living in apartment communities. To combat institutionalization, New York created an extensive congregate housing program (referred to as Enriched Housing) in 1978. Through this program, service coordinators were brought into pre-existing apartment communities to provide necessary services that support the elderly residents. Since then, the state has added numerous other basic service programs in

APPENDIX B (continued)

existing housing, including the Adult Home program, the Personal Care program, and NORC service programs.

In addition, New York's Department of Health created the Assisted Living Program. The Assisted Living Program provides a broad range of services for 4,200 elderly residents of congregate housing in an effort to delay institutionalization. The program provides housing, meals, housekeeping and transportation through SSI and home-based care through Medicaid. Additional services, such as therapy, medication management and intermittent nursing care are available through the program, via private pay.

Older New Yorkers benefit from a wealth of community options. Today, the number of persons living in institutions, primarily nursing homes, in New York has decreased, while the number of seniors living in non-institutional settings has grown faster than the 65 plus population as a whole (U.S. Census Bureau, 2000).

Washington   **It Takes a Village to Age in Place**

Elder Village, Seattle

The Seattle Housing Authority (SHA) is one of 30 housing authorities across the nation participating in HUD's "Moving to New Ways" Demonstration Program. This federal program encourages the development of innovative methods to improve the delivery of affordable housing in order to better meet local needs. Through creative and collaborative financing, SHA combined federal, state and local government funds from a variety of programs: Housing Opportunities for People Everywhere (HOPE VI), Low Income Public Housing, Section 8, New Construction and Moderate Rehabilitation, and the Seattle Senior Housing Program. Along with the government funding, SHA acquired additional financing from their non-profit partners, including the Retirement Housing Foundation, Providence Health Systems, AIDS Housing of Washington, Lutheran Alliance to Create Housing, Low Income Housing Institute and more. Seniors are a primary target population for SHA, which also provides affordable housing to individuals with disabilities, recent immigrants and refugees, families faced with welfare time limits, and low wage earners.

Elder Village combines affordable housing with customized services that allow its senior residents to age in place. It consists of three facilities: (1) Peter Claver House, which has 80 units for completely independent seniors; (2) Esperanza, an 84 unit Section 8 facility with a 24 hour emergency system, counseling and limited services; and (3) Park Place, an assisted living community for 154 frail seniors of which 100 units are designated affordable, using Section 8 vouchers and Medicaid funded services, e.g., medication management, 24 hour on-call RN, LN or LVN nursing staff, housekeeping, meal service, and social activities with social workers and service coordinators on-site. These three facilities are linked to each other by an avenue of shops, a grocery store, nearby transit stops, a clinic with occupational therapists available, senior center for communal activities, a community flower and vegetable garden along with common areas for reading, exercise programs and arts and crafts. The co-location of services at Elder Village promotes effective service delivery to senior residents in need of low-cost housing who want to age in place.

Housing and Services: Provider Examples

Facility/Provider	Programs/ License	Residents	Services Offered	Services: Payment and Provider	Innovative Management
America House MICHIGAN	Section 8, Medicaid waivers, LIHTC	2,813 in 29 facilities	Meals, activities, transportation, health screening, light/heavy housekeeping, personal care	Medicaid waivers, OAA, private pay for a la carte services	Began as a demonstration program; excellent working relationships with local government agencies; residents maintain store to raise funds for activities
Bethany Homes NORTH DAKOTA	Section 202, Section 8, HUD ALCP/ SNF & AL licenses	378	Service coordinator & social worker, meals, activities, health screening, light/heavy housekeeping, personal care, emergency response	Meals and housekeeping a la carte, Medicaid for AL, private pay for SNF	Wellness program: professionals donate dental, podiatry & optometric services to the residents on-site; makes resident families a priority, e.g., encourages family members to visit for meals
Elder Village WASHINGTON	Section 202, Section 8/ Boarding Home license	84	Service coordinator & social workers, meals, activities, health screening, medication management	Medicaid waivers, OAA, Seattle city funds, private pay	Seattle sold land for site below market value; inter-entity management and extensive co-location, with multiple levels of care, clinic, activities, and senior center on site
Fairbanks Pioneer Home ALASKA	State-funded, un-licensed assisted living	92	Meals, activities, transportation, case management, light/heavy housekeeping, personal care, health screening, emergency system	State funds, resident fees	State general fund pays half of costs, residents pay gap; targeting for residents with dementia; extensive use of community volunteers; modified environment
Fowler Christian Apartments TEXAS	Section 202, Section 8, Medicaid waivers/ AL license	139	Service coordinator, lunch, transportation, health screening, housekeeping, personal care	Medicaid, private pay a la carte	First AL pilot program in Texas to be fully funded through HUD and Medicaid

APPENDIX C (continued)

Facility/Provider	Programs/License	Residents	Services Offered	Services: Payment and Provider	Innovative Management
Helen Sawyer Plaza FLORIDA	Section 202/ Extended Congregate Care license	104	Meals, housekeeping, personal care	Medicaid, private pay a la carte	First affordable housing building with licensed assisted living program
Immanuel House CONNECTICUT	Section 236/ Managed Residential Community license	220	Service coordinator, lunch, housekeeping, personal care, medication management	Medicaid, private pay a la carte, services also provided by local hospital and Meals on Wheels	Inter-entity management allows for shared service coordinator and van
Stafford House NEW HAMPSHIRE	Section 8, Section 202, CHSP/ Home Health Care license	90	Meals, day care, personal care, case management, medication management	Medicaid waivers, state funds, private pay a la carte	Extensive resource brokering, e.g., owns adjacent mini-mall & contracts space to hospital for clinic and to meal providers; residents raise funds for additional services
Mid-Peninsula Housing CALIFORNIA	Section 202, Section 8	125	Meals, transportation, health screening, housekeeping, personal care, medication management	Medicaid waiver, corporate sponsors, private pay a la carte	Makes use of wide range of community resources including computer training, ESL, and wellness programs
Penn South Co-op NEW YORK	NORC	1,500	Social day program, comprehensive social and health services	State and city contracts, housing co-op funds, foundations	Contract out 98% of services using partners: VNA, Jewish Home & Hospital
Project New Hope CALIFORNIA	Section 202, Section 8	80	Meals, activities, case management, light/heavy housekeeping, health screening	Medicaid waivers, private pay	Targets seniors with HIV/AIDS; uses outside resources including AngelFood meal program, Jewish Community Center, and Shelter Partnership
The Retreat COLORADO	PACE	55	Extensive PACE service	Medicaid waivers, private pay, insurance	Staff sensitivity training; modified environment; residents may work on sight for discounts

APPENDIX D
Completed Interviews

Linda Adams
Montana
Accessible Space Inc.

Patricia Atkinson
Alaska
Rural Assisted Living Long-Term Care Development Unit

Mandi Birchfield
Texas
Fowler Christian Apartments

Julie Bornstein
California
Keston Infrastructure Institute, University of Southern California

Willard Brown
Washington
Elder Village

William Calderin
Florida
Helen Sawyer Plaza

Sarah Carpenter
Vermont
State Finance Agency

John Carr
California
Department of Aging

Dominique Cohen
California
Mid-Peninsula Housing

Karen Davenport
New Jersey
Robert Wood Johnson Foundation

Karen Dean
Connecticut
Immanuel House

Charlotte DeBois
New Hampshire
Laconia Housing and Redevelopment Authority

Maggie Dionne
Massachusetts
Supportive Housing

Beth Eisenhandler
New York
State Department of Health

Barbara Fuller
New Jersey
Department of Health and Senior Services

APPENDIX D (continued)

Steve Golant
Florida
University of Florida

Karin Hammer-Williamson
Vermont
Department of Aging and Disabilities

Jennie Chin Hansen
California
On Lok Senior Health

Ken Harris
New York
Association of Homes and Services for the Aging

Sylvia Karl
California
Southern California Presbyterian Services

Shelly Kritzman
Michigan
Michigan State Housing Development Authority

Jane Lowe
New Jersey
Robert Wood Johnson Foundation

Deb Macadoo
Vermont
Department of Aging and Disabilities

Jim Maguire
Michigan
1B Area Agency on Aging

Jan Monks
Ohio
American Association of Service Coordinators

Pam Marron
Michigan
American House

Susan Parks
Florida
Housing Finance Corporation

Jack Plimpton
California
Project Hope

Carla Pope
Iowa
Housing Finance Authority

Vera Prosper
New York
State Office on Aging

APPENDIX D (continued)

Charlie Reed
Washington
Homecare Quality Authority

Marty Robb
Massachusetts
Department of Housing and Community Development

Corky Rogers
Colorado
The Retreat

Herb Sanderson
Arkansas
Aging and Adult Services

Nancy Sheehan
Connecticut
University of Connecticut

Diane Sprague
Minnesota
Housing Finance Agency

Alayna Waldrum
California
California Association of Homes and Services for the Aging

Ray Weisgarber
North Dakota
Bethany Homes: Retirement Residence & Skilled Nursing Facility

Vicky Wilson
Alaska
Fairbanks Pioneer Home

Nat Yalowitz
New York
Penn South NORC Social Services

Public Funding
for Long-Term Care Services
for Older People
in Residential Care Settings

Janet O'Keeffe

Joshua Wiener

SUMMARY. State interest in funding residential care through Medicaid is fueled by a desire to offer a full array of home and community-based services (HCBS), reduce nursing home utilization, and achieve the economies of scale of nursing home care without the undesirable institutional characteristics. This paper focuses on state policies–particularly Medicaid policies–that affect access to and the availability and quality of publicly financed residential care for people of limited financial means. *[Article copies available for a fee from The Haworth Document Delivery Service: 1-800-HAWORTH. E-mail address: <docdelivery@haworthpress.com> Website: <http://www.HaworthPress.com> © 2004 by The Haworth Press, Inc. All rights reserved.]*

Janet O'Keeffe, DrPH, RN, and Joshua Wiener, PhD, are affiliated with the RTI International and Information Brokering for Long-Term Care, a project of the Center for Home Care Policy & Research of the Visiting Nurse Service of New York.

The authors wish to thank Penny Hollander Feldman, Joann Ahrens, and the reviewers for their useful comments. The opinions expressed in this paper are those of the authors and do not necessarily reflect the views of RTI International, the Robert Wood Johnson Foundation, or the Visiting Nurse Service of New York.

Funded by the Robert Wood Johnson Foundation.

[Haworth co-indexing entry note]: "Public Funding for Long-Term Care Services for Older People in Residential Care Settings." O'Keeffe, Janet, and Joshua Wiener. Co-published simultaneously in *Journal of Housing for the Elderly* (The Haworth Press, Inc.) Vol. 18, No. 3/4, 2004, pp. 51-79; and: *Linking Housing and Services for Older Adults: Obstacles, Options, and Opportunities* (eds: Jon Pynoos, Penny Hollander Feldman, and Joann Ahrens) The Haworth Press, Inc., 2004, pp. 51-79. Single or multiple copies of this article are available for a fee from The Haworth Document Delivery Service [1-800- HAWORTH, 9:00 a.m. - 5:00 p.m. (EST). E-mail address: docdelivery@haworthpress.com].

KEYWORDS. Long-term care, housing, aging, affordable, public policy, Medicaid, low-income, residential care, assisted living

Objectives

The paper addresses four main questions:

1. How do states use Medicaid to fund services in residential care settings?
2. How do Medicaid's federal rules and state policy choices determine residential care options as well as eligibility for and access to these options?
3. Are Medicaid reimbursement rates and beneficiaries' income adequate to cover costs?
4. How do states assure the quality of care provided to Medicaid beneficiaries in residential care settings and their ability to age in place?

Findings

How do states use Medicaid to fund services in residential care settings?

States have two main options to finance long-term care (LTC) services in residential care settings under the Medicaid program: personal care services provided under the state plan and HCBS provided through a waiver program. By 2002, 40 states and the District of Columbia covered services in residential care settings under Medicaid–27 under HCBS waivers, five under the personal care option, and eight under both options. Each option offers the following advantages and disadvantages:

- Under the personal care option states may serve a less severely impaired population, while under the waiver program beneficiaries must require a nursing home level of care.
- Under the HCBS waiver authority, states can provide services not covered by a state's Medicaid program, such as personal emergency response systems, respite care, and environmental accessibility adaptations, as long as these services are required to keep a person from being institutionalized.
- The waiver authority allows states to limit services to specific counties or regions of a state and to target services to certain groups–strategies that are not normally allowed under Medicaid.

In either case, federal Medicaid rules require that states pay for only the service component of care in a residential care setting. Coverage of room and board costs is permitted only in institutions, such as nursing homes, intermediate care facilities for persons with mental retardation, and hospitals.

How do Medicaid's federal rules and state policy choices determine residential care options, and eligibility for and access to these options?

State policy choices include those related to their Medicaid programs as well as those related to the licensing and regulation of residential care facilities. While state Medicaid programs operate under federal rules, states have considerable flexibility to design their programs by taking advantage of numerous federal options.

Targeting:

- States have considerable discretion to set their own nursing home level-of-care criteria, and these criteria vary widely. Some states require a person to have extensive medical and nursing needs in addition to functional limitations in order to receive nursing home care, whereas other states may require a person to have only functional limitations.
- A state with strict nursing home eligibility standards may choose to cover services in residential care settings through the personal care option in order to extend services to people who do not qualify for nursing home care but who nevertheless need more care than can be safely and cost effectively provided at home.
- To use the waiver program, a state's licensing and regulatory provisions for residential care settings must allow them to serve individuals who meet the state's nursing home level-of-care criteria. Consequently, the residential care options available to individuals with limited means are determined by the complex interplay of Medicaid policy and state licensing and regulatory policy.

Financial Eligibility:

- Waiver programs can increase access by expanding the number of people who are financially eligible for services. Federal law allows states to provide Medicaid waiver services to persons with incomes up to 300 percent of the federal Supplemental Security Income (SSI) payment level, which is the institutional income standard in many states. In 2001, 44 states took advantage of this Medicaid eligibility option, although not all states provided coverage at the maximum allowable level.

Spousal Protection:

- States have the option of providing the spouses of Medicaid waiver clients the same income and asset protections afforded to the community

spouses of persons who reside in nursing homes, which are much more generous than community-based eligibility standards that apply under the personal care option.
- Married couples in states without spousal protection for community care have a financial disincentive to receive waiver services at home or in residential care settings.

Spend Down:

- Medicaid coverage of residential care services can provide a safety net for persons who use their assets to pay privately for residential care. For those who spend down, however, a number of barriers may prevent them from receiving Medicaid services, including:
  - providers who do not accept Medicaid
  - unaffordable room and board charges
  - waiver waiting list
  - not meeting a state's nursing home level-of-care criteria

Licensing:

- With very few exceptions, states do not regulate the name residential care settings use for marketing purposes. Indiscriminate use of the term "assisted living" obscures the differences between types of residential care settings and makes it very difficult for consumers–both private pay and Medicaid eligible–to determine which setting will best meet their current and future needs.

Are Medicaid reimbursement rates and beneficiaries' income adequate to cover costs?

Given the various fiscal constraints on Medicaid programs, state payment rates may be inadequate to attract high quality providers and to assure that sufficient resources are available to provide needed services. No research to date has looked at the adequacy of reimbursement rates; however, the magnitude of differences among maximum payment rates raises concerns that some states may not be paying adequately for services.

Because Medicaid pays for room and board only in institutions, the inability of Medicaid clients to pay for room and board can be a major barrier to increasing the use of residential care for this population. States have several options for making room and board costs affordable for Medicaid clients, including:

1. Limiting the amount providers can charge Medicaid residents for room and board to the federal SSI benefit of $553 minus a small personal needs allowance.
2. Providing a state supplement to the SSI payment for persons living in residential care settings, and limiting the amount that can be charged to the combined SSI plus state supplement payment.
3. Setting waiver clients' maintenance allowance high enough to enable them to pay for room and board.
4. Providing housing subsidies.
5. Permitting family income supplementation.

How do states assure the quality of care provided to Medicaid beneficiaries in residential care settings and their ability to age in place?

Federal Medicaid waiver regulations require participating facilities to meet applicable state standards but do not establish the content of those standards. Thus, assuring the quality of care provided in these settings is almost entirely a state responsibility. State licensing and regulatory provisions cover many areas, including construction and physical plant standards, resident admission and retention standards, staffing, occupancy standards, and health and safety standards.

- Few states require residential care settings receiving Medicaid funding to provide private apartments for Medicaid clients. Many settings provide shared rooms with as many as four residents and shared bathrooms with as many as eight residents.

Staffing and Training:

- Few states establish staffing ratios in residential care settings, preferring to give facilities the flexibility to vary staffing patterns based on the residents' care needs. No consensus exists about the appropriate type and level of staffing needed in residential care settings, particularly nurse staffing. A major problem in reaching such a consensus is that the type and amount of care provided varies significantly across settings, as does the disability level of residents served.
- The type and amount of training provided to staff varies across residential care settings and across states, but for the most part little training is required.
- Determining the appropriate level of licensed nursing services in residential care settings is a contentious issue. Stakeholders disagree on whether these settings should be addressing the needs of very disabled

persons or those with complex medical conditions. Requiring the provision of nursing services would necessitate increases in Medicaid reimbursement rates, which given the fiscal condition of most states are unlikely in the foreseeable future.

Aging in Place:

- Since the inception of the Medicaid program, quality of care systems have been based on the idea that people who need a certain level of care need to be served in particular settings or by particular providers. Allowing residents to age in place requires a different conception of quality assurance than is embedded in the existing regulatory and legal framework.
- Both state regulations and facility policy govern discharge criteria and hence the ability to age in place. All states set restrictions on the type and level of care that can be provided in residential care facilities, primarily through admission and retention criteria. The most common restriction is that people who require a skilled as opposed to an intermediate level of nursing care cannot be served in a residential care setting.
- Giving providers discretion to determine whom they will serve can allow residents to stay in a setting even as their needs increase. It can also lead to both inappropriate retention and inappropriate discharge ("creaming" light care residents).
- The ability to age in place–a key tenet of the assisted living philosophy–is proving very difficult to operationalize. Stakeholders disagree about the extent to which residential care can, or should be expected to, meet the needs of ever more impaired residents requiring increasingly intensive services.

Conclusions

States seeking to make residential care an option for older persons with limited means are grappling with a number of issues that require the reconciliation of what appear to be inherently contradictory goals. These include finding ways to:

- Meet expectations for privacy, amenities, and quality services that have been set by the private pay dominated model of "assisted living" when Medicaid cannot afford to pay private pay rates.
- Cover the actual costs of serving frail older individuals with chronic care needs in residential care settings, when Medicaid is not permitted to pay for room and board and the payment sources available to cover room and board are insufficient.

- Give consumers a sense of what they should reasonably be able to expect from a setting that calls itself "assisted living" or "adult foster care" or some other name, without imposing uniform definitions through state regulation.
- Assure a minimally acceptable quality of care without imposing rules that stifle improvements and without the regulated "floor" becoming the "ceiling."
- Make it possible for individuals to "age in place" without making residential care settings into de facto nursing homes by virtue of having to meet the needs of ever older and more impaired residents.

States need to find the appropriate balance between these goals, which will vary depending on their fiscal and political environment and the unique characteristics of their LTC and residential care systems.

INTRODUCTION

Virtually all individuals who need long-term care (LTC) services prefer to receive them in their own homes, and the majority do so.[1] Nearly two million Americans, however, live in group residential care settings–about half in licensed facilities and half in unlicensed boarding homes.[2] Older people move to group residential care facilities for a variety of reasons:

1. They require unscheduled assistance or 24-hour supervision and do not have sufficient informal care.
2. They cannot afford to pay privately for services in their own homes.
3. They want the social interaction available in these settings, as well as services such as housekeeping, laundry, meals and 24-hour emergency assistance.

This paper focuses on state policies–particularly Medicaid policies–that affect access to and the availability and quality of publicly financed residential care for people of limited financial means. At one time, only a very small portion of Medicaid LTC spending was spent on home and community-based services (HCBS). However, by federal fiscal year 2002, 30 percent of Medicaid LTC spending was for such services, and these outlays are one of the fastest growing components of total Medicaid spending.[3] Coverage of services in residential care has been part of that expansion. Many states hope that these settings will provide more homelike care, provide greater personal autonomy, and cost less than nursing homes do. Moreover, many states contend that these settings provide greater economies of scale than does home care, especially for persons who need a great deal of ongoing supervision, such as persons with Alzheimer's disease.

The first section of the paper provides background information, defining and categorizing the various types of residential care settings and describing the emergence and growth of assisted living as a distinct model of residential care. The paper then addresses four main questions:

1. How do states use Medicaid to fund services in residential care settings?
2. How do Medicaid's federal rules and state policy choices determine residential care options as well as eligibility for and access to these options?
3. Are Medicaid reimbursement rates and beneficiaries' income adequate to cover costs?
4. How do states assure the quality of care provided to Medicaid beneficiaries in residential care settings and the ability of residents to age in place?

The final section of the paper presents our conclusions.

BACKGROUND

Types of Residential Care

Virtually all states license group residential care settings for persons with physical or mental impairments that affect their ability to live independently. States historically have licensed two general types of group residential care: (1) adult foster care, which typically serves five or fewer residents in a provider's home; and (2) congregate care, which typically serves six or more residents in a range of settings (from large residential homes to settings that look like commercial apartment buildings or nursing homes).

More than thirty names are used for licensed residential care facilities including: adult foster care, adult family homes, board and care homes, rest homes, adult care home, domiciliary care homes, personal care homes, community based residential facilities, and assisted living.

Until recently, the most frequently used term for congregate care was board and care, though today all types of congregate care are generally referred to as assisted living.[4,5] The physical character of a substantial portion of congregate care is quite institutional, with two to four persons sharing a bedroom, and as many as eight to ten residents sharing a bathroom.[6]

The Emergence of Assisted Living as a New Model of Care

A new and overlapping model of residential care called assisted living was developed in the late 1980s. The key philosophical tenets of assisted living are based on the goals of meeting residents' needs, promoting independence and dignity, and allowing residents to age in place in a homelike environment. According to three of the major assisted living industry trade associations, privacy and flexible services that will meet residents' needs and allow them to age in place are key elements of the philosophy of assisted living.[7] Many observers view assisted living as a promising LTC model that serves an important role in bridging the "chasm" between receiving care in one's home and in an institution.[8]

The new assisted living model of residential care is popular with older people because it offers what nursing homes and traditional board and care facilities generally do not–privacy and the ability to have greater control over daily activities. Another reason for its popularity is that assisted living facilities built in the 1990s have more desirable physical environments than do board and care facilities and nursing homes, many of which were built in the 1960s and 1970s.

From its beginnings in the U.S. in the late 1980s, through the late 1990s, the assisted living model was the most rapidly growing type of residential care for elderly persons.[9] The major driving forces behind this growth were the actual and projected growth in the elderly population and consumer demand coupled with the ability of a segment of the elderly population to pay out-of-pocket for assisted living, which costs between $26,000 to $36,000 per year.[10] Persons with a high level of need can pay even more.

This paper uses the term "residential care setting" to refer to group residential care generally, and the term "assisted living" to refer to a specific model of care that provides, at a minimum, private rooms and baths (with or without kitchens), and 24-hour staff to assist with scheduled and unscheduled needs.

HOW DO STATES USE MEDICAID TO FUND SERVICES IN RESIDENTIAL CARE SETTINGS?

Given the high cost of the assisted living model, people with limited means will not be able to afford this LTC option without public funding. Prior to the advent of the assisted living model, there was little interest in expanding public funding for residential care for older persons eligible for Medicaid. But with the availability of a "desirable" alternative to nursing homes, many stakeholders–including policy makers, consumer advocacy groups, and providers–have recommended increased Medicaid funding to help subsidize "affordable assisted living" for elderly persons with limited means.[11]

Overview of Medicaid Funding Options[12]

States have two main options to finance LTC services in residential care facilities under the Medicaid program. Since the mid-1970s, they have had the option to offer personal care services as a regular Medicaid state plan service. Personal care provided under the state plan includes help with activities of daily living (ADLs), such as bathing and dressing, and instrumental activities of daily living (IADLs), such as meal preparation. The state plan personal care option does not cover skilled nursing, therapy services, or socialization. Like other Medicaid services, states must offer personal care as an open-ended entitlement–a legal obligation on the part of government to provide services to individuals who meet pre-established criteria, regardless of the cost to the government. In addition, services must be offered on a statewide basis. Only persons financially eligible for Medicaid under the state plan may receive Medicaid-financed personal care services.

In response to the perceived need for coverage of a wider range of HCBS and a desire by states to have greater fiscal control over the expansion of these services, Congress authorized HCBS waivers in 1981. Under Section 1915(c) of the Social Security Act, states may apply to the U.S. Department of Health and Human Services for a waiver of certain federal requirements to allow states to provide HCBS to individuals who would otherwise require services in an institution. Under the HCBS waiver authority, states can provide services not covered by a state's Medicaid program, such as personal emergency response systems, respite care, and environmental accessibility adaptations, as long as these services are required to keep a person from being institutionalized. Additionally, states may provide through a waiver program the same services available through its state plan without the limitations on amount, duration, and scope that apply to these services under the state plan.

The waiver authority allows states to *limit services* to specific counties or regions of a state and to target services to certain groups–strategies that are not normally allowed under Medicaid. In addition, states must establish in advance how many people they will serve during the course of a year. Thus, in contrast to the regular Medicaid program, states may establish waiting lists for these waiver programs. Finally, average expenditures for waiver beneficiaries must be the same or less than they would have been without the waiver (no more than average Medicaid nursing home costs).[13] Importantly, while services may be covered in residential care facilities, room and board may not.

Medicaid can cover room and board only in institutions, such as nursing homes, intermediate care facilities for persons with mental retardation, and hospitals.

From the inception of the waiver program, states have used waivers to pay for services in residential care settings as an alternative to intermediate care facilities for persons with mental retardation (ICF/MRs). In 1981 Oregon became the first state to use the Medicaid waiver program to cover services in residential care settings for elderly persons, but few states other than Oregon used waivers to pay for residential care services for the elderly population until the 1990s. From 1998 to 2000, however, the number of Medicaid beneficiaries receiving LTC services in group residential settings outside of nursing homes increased by 46 percent to 58,544 beneficiaries.[14] From 2000 to 2002, the number increased by 75 percent to 102,000 beneficiaries (see Chart 1).[15]

By 2002, 40 states and the District of Columbia covered services in residential care facilities under Medicaid; 27 under HCBS waivers, five under the personal care option, and eight under both options (see Table 1).[16]

HOW DO MEDICAID'S FEDERAL RULES AND STATE POLICY CHOICES DETERMINE RESIDENTIAL CARE OPTIONS AND ELIGIBILITY FOR AND ACCESS TO THESE OPTIONS?

States' policy choices include those related to their Medicaid program as well as those related to the licensing and regulation of residential care settings. While state Medicaid programs operate under federal rules, states nevertheless have considerable flexibility to design their programs. The combination of federal rules and state policy choices affects which residential care options are available, as well as eligibility for and access to residential care settings.

CHART 1. Medicaid Beneficiaries Receiving LTC in Group Residential Services Outside of Nursing Homes

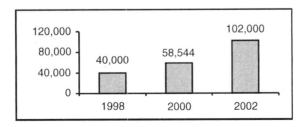

TABLE 1. States Using Medicaid to Cover Services in Residential Care Facilities

Waiver (27)		Personal Care (5)	Waiver and Personal Care (8)
Alaska	Montana	Massachusetts	Arkansas
Arizona	Nebraska	Missouri	Florida
Colorado	Nevada	New York	Idaho
Connecticut	New Hampshire	North Carolina	Maine
Delaware	New Jersey	South Carolina	Michigan
District of Columbia	New Mexico		Minnesota
Georgia	Oregon		Vermont
Hawaii	Pennsylvania		Wisconsin
Illinois	Rhode Island		
Indiana	South Dakota		
Iowa	Texas		
Kansas	Washington		
Maryland	Wyoming		
Mississippi			

Targeting by Functional Criteria

A state's decision as to which Medicaid option to use–personal care, waiver, or both–is based in large part on the state's current LTC system and its policy goals. Using the personal care option can increase access by broadening eligibility to serve a less severely impaired population because, unlike the waiver, states may cover persons who do not require a nursing home level of care. On the other hand, if the state wants to target a narrower population, then the waiver is the appropriate choice because eligibility is limited to people who are nursing home eligible.[17]

Within federal Medicaid guidelines, states have considerable discretion to set their own nursing home level-of-care criteria, and these criteria vary widely. Some states require a person to have extensive medical and nursing needs in addition to functional limitations in order to receive nursing home care, whereas other states may require a person to have only functional limitations. Thus, as with many other parts of the Medicaid program, depending on the state where they live, persons with the same level of need may have very different options.[18]

A state with strict nursing home eligibility standards may choose to cover services in residential care settings through the personal care option in order to extend services to people who do not qualify for nursing home care, but who nevertheless need more care than can be safely and cost effectively provided at home. Massachusetts, for example, uses the state plan to provide personal care services to people who are frail but not nursing home eligible.[19] Massachusetts covers up to two hours of personal care and associated administrative expenses through the personal care option to Medicaid beneficiaries in Group Adult Foster Care.[20] Massachusetts also created a special SSI supplement specifically for eligible residents to help them pay for room and board.[21]

To use the waiver program, a state's licensing and regulatory provisions for residential care settings must allow them to serve individuals who meet the state's nursing home level-of-care criteria. Consequently, the residential care options available to individuals with limited means are determined by the complex interplay of Medicaid policy and state licensing and regulatory policy. States that serve clients with a high level of need through their personal care program may be providing a viable residential care option for some Medicaid clients who in other states might be served through the waiver program, but the personal care option is restricted to those who meet the more stringent financial eligibility criteria for state plan services.

Financial Eligibility

Waiver programs can increase access by expanding the number of people who are financially eligible for services. Federal law allows states to provide Medicaid waiver services to persons with incomes up to 300 percent of the federal Supplemental Security Income (SSI) payment level, which is the institutional income standard in many states. In 2001, 44 states took advantage of this Medicaid eligibility option, although not all states provided coverage at the maximum allowable level.[22]

In contrast, to be eligible for personal care under the state plan, individuals must meet usual community-based eligibility standards, which (depending on the state) are: (1) the SSI level, (2) up to 100 percent of the federal poverty level, or (3) the state's medically needy income standard. The higher eligibility standard in the waiver programs is designed to "level the playing field" between institutional and non-institutional services.

Spousal Protections

States have the option of providing the spouses of Medicaid waiver clients the same income and asset protections afforded to the community spouses of persons who reside in nursing homes, which are much more generous than community-based eligibility standards that apply under the personal care option. In 2001, the level of protected assets for community-based aged, blind and disabled Medicaid beneficiaries was usually around $2,000, but varied from $17,400 to $87,000 for the spouses of nursing home residents. During that year, 38 states and the District of Columbia had adopted the nursing home spousal impoverishment rules for spouses of waiver beneficiaries, while 13 states had not.[23]

Married couples in states without spousal protection for community care have a financial disincentive to receive waiver services at home or in residential care settings. For example, some nursing home residents in Florida who wanted to transition to a residential care setting were reportedly unwilling to do so because the move would impoverish their spouses.[24]

Spend Down

Residential care can be expensive. A national survey of facilities conducted by RTI International in 1998 found that while basic rates ranged from $16,000 to $26,000 per year, persons seeking high privacy and service levels can expect to pay about 30 percent more.[25] Based on older persons' income, the study concluded that only a third of persons 65 and older could afford even the most common basic annual rate of about $19,000. However, in 1996, 40 percent of the population age 75 and older had assets between $171,000 and $485,000, and there is reason to believe that many elderly persons in assisted living are using assets to pay for residential care.[26] One study of assisted living residents found that over 60 percent had incomes less than $25,000, and concluded that while some received financial help from family, most moderate and lower-income residents are paying for market rate assisted living by spending down their assets–primarily from the sale of a home.[27]

Medicaid coverage of residential care services can provide a safety net for persons who use their assets to pay privately for residential care. For those who spend down, however, a number of barriers may prevent them from receiving Medicaid services:

1. *Not all settings accept Medicaid.* Some may not admit new Medicaid eligible residents but will allow long-stay residents who spend down to continue to reside in the facility. If a facility does not accept Medicaid under any condition, a person who spends down will have to move (and may not be able to find a setting within traveling distance of family or friends).
2. *Not all states limit the amount that providers can charge Medicaid residents for room and board.* Consequently, individuals may exhaust their assets in a facility that accepts Medicaid service payments, but be unable to afford room and board. Persons who have spent down and cannot afford to pay for room and board will have to find a facility that both accepts Medicaid and has affordable room and board charges.
3. *Individuals may spend down in a facility that accepts Medicaid and is affordable, but still not be able to receive services because there is no*

waiver "slot" available. Many states control expenditures by limiting the number of persons who can be served through the waiver, which often results in waiting lists for waiver services.[28] States are reluctant to expand the number of waiver slots when someone spends down to eligibility in residential care because this would create an entitlement to waiver services for people in residential care. Moreover, over time, this could result in a higher proportion of waiver funds going to residential care than to people residing in their own homes, which is considered undesirable by some states. In Wisconsin, for example, some counties are reluctant to spend limited waiver funds on residential care, which they view as "quasi-institutional" settings.[29]

4. *A person may spend down to Medicaid financial eligibility and not meet the state's nursing home level-of-care criteria.* In such a case, the person will be ineligible for the waiver program and will have to find a residential care setting that will both provide the level of care needed and accept what he or she can afford to pay.

State Licensing Provisions and Residential Care Options

Residential care settings are governed almost exclusively by state laws and regulations, rather than by federal rules, and vary from state to state.[30] With very few exceptions, however, states do not regulate the names used by residential care settings. Due to the popularity of assisted living, virtually all residential care settings market themselves as assisted living even though they have markedly different physical environments, service packages, and amenities. Under pressure from the residential care industry some states have amended their statutes to rename domiciliary care homes, board and care homes, and even adult foster care, as assisted living.

Indiscriminate use of the term assisted living obscures the differences between types of residential care settings, and makes it very difficult for consumers–both private pay and Medicaid eligible–to determine which setting will best meet their current and future needs. Representatives of the residential care industry oppose prescriptive regulatory requirements for "assisted living" (such as requiring private rooms) because they contend it will prevent providers from offering a variety of physical settings and service packages, thereby reducing consumer choice.[31] But creating regulatory requirements for a particular model of care called assisted living does not prevent providers from offering other types of care, it only prevents providers from calling these other types of care assisted living. Due to the popularity of the new model of assisted living, however, providers fear they will be put at a competitive disadvantage if they cannot market themselves as assisted living.[32]

With few exceptions, such as Oregon, states are not addressing this issue. Consequently, group residential care for elderly persons has become the "black box" of LTC services. Consumers have a general understanding of what to expect in home care and nursing home care, but not in residential care. In a recent study of six states' use of Medicaid to fund services in residential care settings, stakeholders in every state except Oregon cited public confusion about residential care options as a major problem.[33] In the words of one state ombudsman, "people don't have a clue; they think that assisted living provides everything a nursing home does, but a la carte and in nicer surroundings."[34]

ARE MEDICAID REIMBURSEMENT RATES AND BENEFICIARIES' INCOME ADEQUATE TO COVER COSTS?

Given the various fiscal constraints on Medicaid programs, states generally do not pay market rates for services in residential care settings, raising concerns about whether payments are adequate to meet residents' care needs.

Service Payments

Adequate payment rates are critical to attract high quality providers and to assure that sufficient resources are available to provide needed services.[35] States paying for a broad range of services under a waiver use a variety of payment methods, including flat rates, tiered rates, case-mix rates, and fee-for-service rates.[36] Thirteen states use flat rates, where all providers receive the same payment rate without adjustment for case mix. This payment methodology creates incentives to admit residents who need less care and to discharge residents when their service needs become too costly, which decreases the likelihood that residents can age in place. Tiered, case-mix-adjusted, and fee-for-service rates create incentives to serve more impaired residents because additional services or higher levels of disability lead to more reimbursement.

As noted earlier, under federal rules for HCBS waivers, Medicaid costs for persons in residential care settings cannot exceed the nursing home costs that would have been incurred in the absence of the waiver. States can use either a fixed per capita amount for each beneficiary or they can average expenditures across waiver beneficiaries. The latter method provides more flexibility because it allows some beneficiaries to exceed the nursing facility cost as long as costs for others in the program are lower and the average waiver cost does not exceed the average nursing facility cost. States also have the option of setting the waiver payment cap at a percentage of nursing home costs, e.g., 80 percent. Maximum monthly waiver rates for services in residential care settings vary considerably among states, from $840 in Florida to $3,987 in Minnesota.

States that cover residential care services through the personal care option typically cover a less severely impaired population than those eligible for waiver services and cover only a small amount of personal care.[37] For example, North Carolina pays for one hour of care per day in residential care settings.[38] Consequently, Medicaid personal care payments are typically much less than waiver payments. Florida uses both Medicaid options and pays $278 a month ($9.28 a day) for personal care services provided under the state plan, compared to $840 a month ($28 a day) for waiver services provided in residential care settings.

No research to date has looked at the adequacy of reimbursement rates. Nonetheless, the magnitude of differences among maximum payment rates raises concerns that some states may not be paying adequately for services. Furthermore, inadequate payment for services may be compounded by state-imposed restrictions on what providers can charge Medicaid residents for room and board. While such restrictions, which are discussed below, are usually imposed to make residential care more affordable for Medicaid clients, when combined with low service payments they could have the perverse effect of reducing access by deterring providers from serving the Medicaid market.

Adequacy of Private Funds for Room and Board

As noted earlier, Medicaid pays for room and board only in institutions. Thus, *the inability of Medicaid clients to pay for room and board can be a major barrier to increasing access to residential care for this population.*[39] States have employed the following range of additional options to make room and board costs affordable for Medicaid clients.

1. *Limit the amount facilities can charge Medicaid clients for room and board to the federal SSI benefit, which in 2003 was $553 minus a small personal needs allowance.*[40]
2. *Provide a state supplement to the SSI payment for persons living in residential care settings, and limit the amount that can be charged to the combined SSI plus state supplement payment.* State supplements vary from negligible ($1.70 in Oregon) to substantial ($560 in North Carolina).[41] Of the 28 states that have a supplement, 21 provide less than $100 a month.[42]
3. *Set the Medicaid personal maintenance allowance high enough to pay for room and board.* Persons eligible for the waiver under the 300 percent of SSI income eligibility rule may have incomes up to $1,656 per month. However, not all of this income is available to pay for room and board because waiver clients are required to contribute toward the cost of services. States, at their option, can disregard a certain amount of income that the waiver beneficiary can use to pay for room and board. This amount is typically called a personal maintenance allowance. States vary in the amount of the maintenance allowance they allow, from $800 to $1,656 (the full 300 percent of SSI standard).[43] Not all

waiver clients, however, are eligible under the 300 percent of SSI income rule. Some are SSI eligible, and will have only $553 per month to spend on room and board (minus a small personal needs allowance, typically around $35).

4. *Provide housing subsidies for low-income persons.* Many states are exploring ways to combine Medicaid funding and subsidized housing to create affordable assisted living. Housing subsidies are available through a number of options:

- Low Income Housing Tax Credits
- HUD Section 202 Assisted Living Conversion Program
- Section 8 Rental Assistance Vouchers
- HUD Fair Housing Act Section 232 Mortgage Insurance Program
- Federal Home Loan Bank Affordable Housing Program
- Low Interest Bonds
- U.S. Department of Agriculture Housing Services Programs
- Community Reinvestment Act
- State, City, and other Local Programs.[44]

Typically, multiple public programs are needed to provide an adequate housing subsidy. For example, one affordable assisted living development in Vermont was financed by a combination of funds from HUD's Section 202 Assisted Living Conversion Program, the Vermont Housing and Conservation Board, the Community Development Block Grant and City Trust, HUD Special Purpose Funding, and tax exempt bond financing through the Vermont Housing Agency. However, because housing subsidy programs and Medicaid operate under different requirements, including eligibility rules, extensive planning and collaboration is needed to enable multiple programs to work together.[47]

5. *Allow family supplementation to increase the funds available for room and board, particularly to pay the difference in cost between a shared and a private room.* Family supplementation is considered income in determining eligibility for SSI and may be considered in determining eligibility for Medicaid waiver services, at the state's option, in accordance with SSI rules.[48] Some observers believe that third party supplementation should be allowed because it can improve the quality of life by paying for a private room. Others believe that allowing supplementation will lead to a two-tiered system of care: one for residents whose families can supplement and one for those whose families cannot. In 2002, 19 states permitted family supplementation, 7 prohibited it, and the remainder had either no policy or did not cover services in residential care settings under Medicaid (see Table 2).[49]

TABLE 2. State Policies on Family Supplementation[45]

Allow Supplementation (19)		Prohibit Supplementation (7)	No Policy (4)
Alaska	Montana	Colorado	Missouri
Arizona	Nevada	Delaware	Nebraska
Connecticut	New Jersey	Hawaii	New Hampshire
Florida	New Mexico	Illinois	Washington
Georgia	New York	Maine	
Idaho	North Carolina*	Maryland	
Iowa	Rhode Island	Oregon	
Kansas	South Dakota		
Michigan	Texas		
	Wisconsin		

*North Carolina currently permits family supplementation to pay the difference between the cost of a private and shared room without jeopardizing Medicaid eligibility, but only for people who have spent down in a nursing home. Residential care providers are lobbying the state to allow family supplementation for Medicaid residents in their facilities.[46]

Few states require residential care settings receiving Medicaid funding to provide private apartments or rooms for Medicaid clients. Approximately 40 percent of Medicaid clients in residential care settings receive personal care services through the Medicaid state plan in board and care homes. States permit these facilities to provide shared rooms with as many as four residents and shared bathrooms with as many as eight residents. Thus for many if not most Medicaid beneficiaries, residential care does not afford the privacy that is the hallmark of market-rate assisted living.

HOW DO STATES ASSURE THE QUALITY OF CARE PROVIDED TO MEDICAID BENEFICIARIES IN RESIDENTIAL CARE SETTINGS AND THEIR ABILITY TO AGE IN PLACE?

Federal Medicaid waiver regulations require participating facilities to meet applicable state standards but do not establish the content of those standards, thus assuring that the quality of care provided in residential care settings is almost entirely a state responsibility.[50] State licensing and regulatory provisions cover many areas, including construction and physical plant standards, resident admission and retention standards, staffing, occupancy standards, and health and safety standards.

Staffing

Staffing is a key component of quality of care in residential care settings. In two studies, residential care residents and their families cited staff knowledge and training, staff type, and staffing levels as key elements of the quality of care.[51] Few states require staffing ratios in residential care settings, preferring to give facilities the flexibility to vary staffing patterns based on the residents' care needs.[52]

One study of the assisted living industry in four states found a problem with insufficient, inadequate, and untrained staff.[53] A national survey of residential care facility staff in 1998 found that 58 percent of residents reported that adequate staff was not always available. Additionally, a significant number of staff were poorly informed about some issues related to the care of individuals with dementia, and the majority of staff were almost completely unaware of what constitutes normal aging.[54] The authors concluded that the lack of knowledge of normal aging boded poorly for the early recognition and treatment of relatively common conditions that can often be resolved with treatment.[55]

In a recent study of six states that use Medicaid to pay for services in residential care settings, stakeholders in each of the states expressed concerns about the quality of care in residential care settings mostly due to perceptions of insufficient and untrained staff. Respondents cited inadequate staffing levels in particular, noting that even with highly trained competent staff, insufficient staffing will compromise the quality of care.[56] Finally, articles in the general media have raised concerns about inadequate staffing in residential care settings.[57]

No consensus exists about the appropriate type and level of staffing needed in residential care settings, particularly nurse staffing. A major problem in reaching such a consensus is that the type and amount of care provided varies significantly across settings, as does the disability level and health care needs of the residents.

Nursing and Health Related Services

A major staffing issue for many stakeholders is the appropriate level of licensed nursing services in residential care settings and staff ability to recognize and address health problems. Some experts contend that these settings cannot and should not be expected to meet the needs of persons with a high level of disability and/or medically complex conditions. Similarly, some providers, state officials, and consumer advocates argue that residential care should be a social model of care and having nurses on staff is not only unnecessary but undesirable.[58] On the other hand, some consumer advocates believe that in order to allow residents to age in place, residential care settings need to be able to meet their nursing and health related needs. Depending on a state's nursing home level-of-care criteria, Medicaid residents served through the waiver program may well need a significant amount of skilled nursing services and oversight.

While some stakeholders believe that a higher level of nursing services is needed, they recognize that requiring the provision of nursing services and additional staff training will necessitate increases in Medicaid reimbursement rates. Given most states' budget crises, such increases are unlikely, at least in the foreseeable future.

Training

The type and amount of training provided to staff vary across residential care settings and across states, but for the most part little training is required.[59] Training requirements for providers serving persons with dementia tend to be more specific than those for residential care residents generally.[60] Twenty-eight states have staff training requirements for facilities that serve people with dementia, but in some states they are quite minimal. For example, Nevada requires that within three months of employment direct care staff receive eight hours of training about care provision for residents with dementia. Some states specify topics that must be covered in training, such as common behaviors and recommended behavior management, but not the number of hours required; others specify both topics and hours.[61]

Aging in Place

One of the attractive philosophical tenets of assisted living is the notion of aging in place–meaning that as individuals age and become more disabled, additional services can be provided so that they will not have to move to another residential setting, or to a nursing home. Making aging in place a reality, however, requires a different conception of quality assurance than is embedded in the existing regulatory and legal framework.

Since the inception of the Medicaid program, quality of care systems have been based on the idea that people who need a certain level of care need to be served in particular settings or by particular providers. Individuals with slight disabilities could be cared for at home, and as they became more disabled, they would move to residential care and then to a nursing home. Each level of care would serve individuals with specific types and levels of severity. This idea is operationalized in some states' nursing home eligibility criteria, which define eligibility for nursing home care simply as the need for the type or level of care provided in nursing homes.[62]

When Medicaid began paying for HCBS for nursing home-eligible persons, the assumption that persons who met nursing home eligibility criteria could only be served in a nursing home was challenged. States wanted to be able to serve at least some nursing home-eligible individuals in more homelike settings, but they are still grappling with the question of how to assure quality of care for this population without imposing the regulatory structure found in nursing homes.

The ability of residential care staff to meet high levels of resident need largely determines whether a person can "age in place." Both state regulations and facility policy govern discharge criteria and, hence, the ability to age in place.[63] All states set restrictions on the type and level of care that can be provided in residential care facilities, primarily through admission and retention regulatory criteria. The most common restriction is that people who require a skilled as opposed to an intermediate level of nursing care cannot be served in a residential care setting.

Although OBRA '87 abolished the distinction between intermediate and skilled nursing facilities (SNFs), states were required to continue providing both levels of care within a single nursing facility to Medicaid residents. The former intermediate level-of-care criteria are the minimum level-of-care criteria that a person must meet to be eligible for Medicaid coverage. Individuals who meet this level of care are more likely candidates for waiver services, whether provided in the home or in a residential care setting, than those who need a skilled level-of-care. Skilled nursing facility level-of-care criteria generally require an individual to need skilled services on a daily basis. For example, Michigan's rules governing homes for the aged do not allow anyone who requires intensive nursing care or nursing care on a 24-hour basis to be served in these facilities.[64]

States have different approaches for regulating the provision of services in residential care settings. One approach is to mandate a maximum amount of hours of care that can be provided. For example, in Wisconsin, Residential Care Apartment Complexes are prohibited from retaining any resident who needs more than 28 hours of care per week, including nursing care. On the other hand, Community Based Residential Facilities are prohibited from retaining any resident who needs more than three hours of nursing care a day, but face no restriction on the amount of personal care that can be provided.

Another approach is to identify specific conditions that are not allowed in a given setting, such as severe pressure ulcers or ventilator dependency. A third approach sets a minimum amount of care that must be furnished, and providers are permitted to set their own maximums, based on their ability to meet the needs of a given resident.[65] For example, a provider may feel that current staff can handle one or two heavy care residents but no more than that. Oregon uses this approach, which is based on the premise that individuals should not have to enter a nursing home to receive a specific level of care. However, while its intent is to allow people to stay in a setting even if their needs increase, it can lead to both inappropriate retention and inappropriate discharge. In the former case, a provider may retain residents whose needs exceed a setting's ability to meet them in order to keep occupancy levels high. In the latter case, a provider may "cream" residents by discharging heavy care residents even though the provider can meet their needs.

Beyond state rules regarding the minimum and maximum services that must or may be provided, a facility can set its own policies regarding whom it will serve. For example, a facility may choose not to serve residents who wander or who have other behavioral problems, while another may choose to provide whatever services are needed as long as the resident can pay for them. Some observers argue that residential care facilities cannot be expected to meet the needs of ever more impaired residents without making them into de facto nursing homes, and if they are nursing homes, then they should meet nursing home regulatory standards. In sum, the ability to age in place–a key tenet of the assisted living philosophy–is proving very difficult to operationalize.

CONCLUSIONS

Many states are using Medicaid to expand the use of residential care settings to serve older people with disabilities. They are attracted to residential care settings by the economies of scale that are lacking in traditional HCBS. States hope to promote residential settings that are more homelike, provide greater personal autonomy and privacy, and cost less than nursing homes. In particular, states see potential in residential care settings for people with dementia who need a lot of supervision but not a great deal of medical care. This review of states' use of Medicaid to fund services in residential care settings suggests four overarching policy questions and related trade-offs.

First, should states wanting to expand residential care under Medicaid use the personal care option, HCBS waivers, or both? These choices are consequential to the amount of services provided and who may be eligible. Under the personal care option, states may serve people with modest disability levels, but cannot expand financial eligibility to a broader population and must fund a relatively narrow set of services. Under Medicaid HCBS waivers, states must limit eligibility to people with a nursing home level of care, but may expand financial eligibility and may finance a very broad set of services.

Second, are room and board payments and Medicaid service reimbursement rates adequate to provide good quality care? To assure access for Medicaid beneficiaries, room and board charges must be affordable. States have several options to ensure this, including limiting the amount that providers can charge Medicaid clients to the SSI payment plus state supplement level. However, if states choose this option, they must pay a sufficient amount for services, because it is unlikely that the SSI payment of $552 per month is adequate to cover room and board. Failure to assure that the combination of service payment and room and board payments are adequate may make it difficult to attract high quality providers and to assure that resources are available to provide needed care. Unless payments are at a level that good quality providers will accept, Medicaid beneficiaries may be either unable to find service providers or they will have to utilize a substandard provider. Some analysts have noted that although 40 states now cover services in residential care settings under Medicaid, participation is low, particularly in waiver programs, in part because public payments have lagged behind private-pay rates. Given the fiscal status of most states, significantly higher reimbursement rates are unlikely.

Third, does the existing supply of residential care facilities provide the autonomy and privacy on which the expansion of Medicaid coverage is premised? Many facilities currently participating in Medicaid are board and care homes that have been renamed "assisted living," but lack the philosophical and physical plant characteristics of facilities serving private pay residents. Substantial portions of Medicaid beneficiaries reside in facilities where they must share rooms and bathrooms, just as in nursing facilities. While some states, such as Oregon and Washington, hold Medicaid-participating facilities to higher standards than state licensing rules, most states do not. Because of the enormous variability that exists among residential care providers in the type and amount of services provided, in admission and retention policies, and in the degree of privacy offered, it is not clear that residential care is in fact "better" than nursing homes, particularly for individuals who need a nursing home level of care.

Fourth, how should facilities be regulated to assure adequate quality yet allow older people to age in place? In most cases, current state standards are minimal and vague. While many persons in assisted living have relatively light long-term care and medical needs, a significant minority are quite severely disabled. The use of Medicaid HCBS waivers complicates this question because eligibility is limited to persons with disabilities who need a nursing home level of care. The difficulty is that federal and state regulatory structures are built on the concept of a continuum of care in which individuals move from one level to another as they become more disabled. In contrast, the whole notion of aging in place means bringing services to individuals in their "homes," wherever they may be, as they become more disabled. The issue is how to allow aging in place without making these facilities into unlicensed nursing homes. States are struggling with this issue, without a great deal of consensus on how to proceed. Moreover, no published research has quantitatively studied whether quality of care and quality of life are better in residential care settings than in nursing homes.

In sum, states seeking to make residential care an option for older persons with limited means are grappling with a number of issues that require the reconciliation of what appear to be inherently contradictory goals. These include finding ways to:

- Meet expectations for privacy, amenities, and quality services that have been set by the private pay dominated model of "assisted living" when Medicaid cannot afford to pay private pay rates.
- Cover the actual costs of serving frail older individuals with chronic care needs in residential care settings, when Medicaid is not permitted to pay for room and board and the payment sources available to cover room and board are insufficient.
- Give consumers a sense of what they should reasonably be able to expect from a setting that calls itself "assisted living" or "adult foster care" or some other name, without imposing uniform definitions through state regulation.
- Assure a minimally acceptable quality of care without imposing rules that stifle improvements and without the regulated "floor" becoming the "ceiling."
- Make it possible for individuals to "age in place" without making residential care settings into de facto nursing homes by virtue of having to meet the needs of ever older and more impaired residents.

States need to find the appropriate balance between these goals, which will vary depending on their fiscal and political environment and the unique characteristics of their LTC and residential care systems.

NOTES

1. Mattimore, T.J. et al. "Surrogate and Physician Understanding of Patients' Preferences for Living Permanently in a Nursing Home," *Journal of the American Geriatrics Society* 45, 818-824, 1997; Zinn, J.S., Lavizzo-Mourey, R., and Taylor, L. "Measuring Satisfaction with Care in the Nursing Home Setting: The Nursing Home Resident Satisfaction Scale." *Journal of Applied Gerontology.* 12, 452-465, 1993; AARP, "*Beyond 50.03: A Report to the Nation on Independent Living and Disability,*" Washington, DC, 2003.

2. Newcomer, R. and Maynard, R. (2002). *Residential Care for the Elderly: Supply, Demand, and Quality Assurance.* The California HealthCare Foundation.

3. Burwell, B., Sredl, K., and Eiken, S., *Medicaid Long-Term Care Expenditures in FY 2002,* The MEDSTAT Group, Memorandum, May 13, 2003.

4. Mollica, R. (2002). *State Assisted Living Policy: 2002.* National Academy for State Health Policy, Portland, Maine.

5. Hawes, C., Rose, M., and Phillips, C.D. (December 1999). *A National Study of Assisted Living for the Frail Elderly: Results of a National Survey of Facilities.* U.S. Department of Health and Human Services, Assistant Secretary for Planning and Evaluation, Office of Disability, Aging and Long Term Care Policy.

6. Mollica, R. 2002. op. cit.

7. Hawes, C. (2001). "Introduction," in Zimmerman, S., Sloan, P.D., and Eckert, K. (Eds.) *Assisted Living: Needs, Practices, and Policies in Residential Care for the Elderly.* Baltimore: The Johns Hopkins University Press.

8. Ibid.

9. Hawes, C. et al. (December 1999). op.cit.

10. Hawes, C. et al. (December 1999). op.cit.

11. Assisted Living Workgroup (April 2003). *Assuring Quality in Assisted Living: Guidelines for Federal and State Policy, State Regulations, and Operation.* A Report to the U.S. Senate Special Committee on Aging.

12. This section draws heavily on Chapter Five in Smith, G., O'Keeffe, J. et al. *Understanding Medicaid Home and Community Services: A Primer.* (October 2000.) U.S. Department of Health and Human Services, Office of the Assistant Secretary for Planning and Evaluation.

13. States can use either a fixed per capita amount for each beneficiary or they can average expenditures across waiver beneficiaries. The latter method provides more flexibility because it allows some beneficiaries to exceed the nursing facility cost as long as costs for others in the program are lower and the average waiver cost does not exceed the average nursing facility cost. States have the option of setting the waiver cap at a percentage of nursing home costs, e.g., 80 percent.

14. Mollica, R. (1998). *State Assisted Living Policy: 1998.* National Academy for State Health Policy, Portland, Maine. Mollica, R. (2002). op. cit. In 1998, approximately half of the 40,000 Medicaid beneficiaries were in North Carolina, which provides an hour of personal care per day to residents of adult care homes, through the Medicaid personal care option.

15. Mollica, R. (2002). op. cit.

16. Mollica, R. (2002). op. cit.

17. Personal care is a single service and functional eligibility standards generally reference the need for assistance with ADLs and IADLs only. On the other hand, nursing homes provide multiple services, and waiver programs can provide any service needed to prevent institutionalization.

18. O'Keeffe, J. (December 1996). *Determining the Need for Long-Term Care Services: An Analysis of Health and Functional Eligibility Criteria in Medicaid Home and Community Based Waiver Programs.* Washington, D.C.: AARP.

19. Mollica, R. (2002). op. cit.

20. GAFC residents are also eligible for adult day health center services up to two days a week, and for home health aide services up to eight hours a week. Gulyas, R. (2002). *How States Have Created Affordable Assisted Living: What Advocates and Policy Makers Need to Know.* Washington, D.C.: AARP.

21. In 2000, the supplement was $454 per month. Providers serving GAFC residents who are eligible for the supplement would receive about $2000 a month ($1037 from Medicaid for services, and $966 from the resident for room and board [SSI + supplement.]

22. Bruen, B., Wiener, J., and Thomas, S. (2003). *Medicaid Eligibility for Aged, Blind and Disabled Beneficiaries.* Washington, DC: AARP.

23. Ibid.

24. O'Keeffe, J., O'Keeffe, C., and Bernard, S. (July 2003). *Using Medicaid to Cover Services for Elderly Persons in Residential Care Settings: State Policy Maker and Stakeholder Views in Six States.* U.S. Department of Health and Human Services, Office of the Assistant Secretary for Planning and Evaluation.

25. Facilities can have either a single rate, or multiple rates. Facilities with multiple rates have a base rate which includes a limited amount of services, and charge more for services not covered in the base rate. Hawes, C. et al. (December 1999). op.cit.

26. Newcomer, R., and Maynard, R. (2002). op.cit. Hawes, C. et al. (December 1999). op.cit.

27. *National Survey of Assisted Living Residents: Who Is the Customer?* (1998). Annapolis, MD: National Investment Conference.

28. Wiener, J., Tilly J., and Alecxih, L.M.B., "HCBS for Older Persons and Younger Adults with Disabilities in Seven States," *Health Care Financing Review,* 23(3): 89-114, 2002.

29. O'Keeffe, J. et al. (July 2003). op.cit.

30. No applicable federal statutes exist, other than the Keys Amendment to the Social Security Act, which is applicable to board and care facilities in which a "substantial number of SSI recipients" are likely to reside. However, the Keys amendment is virtually unused to address quality. General Accounting Office. (1989). *Board and Care: Insufficient Assurances that Residents' Needs Are Identified and Met.* Washington, D.C.

31. O'Keeffe, J. et al. (July 2003). op.cit.

32. Ironically, providers' fear of being put at a competitive disadvantage if they cannot market themselves as assisted living has led to situations where the residential care setting that most closely adheres to the assisted living philosophy is not called assisted living. For example, Wisconsin created a new licensure category called assisted living, which required private apartments. Community based residential facilities that do not offer private apartments lobbied the state to allow them to also market themselves as assisted living. Wisconsin revised the statute to allow them to do so and renamed the licensing category of the apartment model to Residential Care Apartment Complex to address concerns that the public would be confused if the new apartment model and community-based residential facilities were both called assisted living.

33. O'Keeffe, J. et al. (July 2003). op.cit.

34. O'Keeffe, J. et al. (July 2003). op.cit.

35. Richard Ladd, personal communication, May 2003.

36. Tiered rates are similar to case mix rates, but typically have only two or three tiers. Case mix rates, on the other hand, can have 14 or more levels.

37. States' nursing home eligibility criteria vary considerably and a person who meets the criteria in one state may not meet it in another. As a result, in some states, some of the people eligible for personal care in one state might be more severely impaired than waiver clients in another state. O'Keeffe, J. (December 1996). op.cit.

38. States offering the personal care option to persons in their own home typically cover a greater number of hours. The minimal amount covered in personal care homes is based on the expectation that these homes are already covering some of the services covered under the personal care option, such as meal preparation.

39. Mollica, R. (2002). op.cit.

40. Mollica, R. (2002). op.cit. Information on the number of states that limit room and board costs to SSI or SSI plus the state supplement is not available.

41. The state's SSI supplement of $1.70 per month was the minimum amount required by federal law as the state's maintenance of effort when the SSI program was first enacted in the early 1970's. O'Keeffe, J. et al. (July 2003). op.cit.

42. Stone, J.L. (2002). *Medicaid: Eligibility for the Aged and Disabled.* Congressional Research Services. Report prepared for Members and Committees of Congress.

43. Robert Mollica, personal communication, December, 2003.

44. Gulyas, R. (2002). op. cit.

45. Mollica, R. (2002). op.cit. Information about family supplementation was not available for all states.

46. O'Keeffe, J. et al. (July 2003) op.cit.

47. Smith, G., O'Keeffe, J. et al. *Understanding Medicaid Home and Community Services: A Primer.* (October 2000). U.S. Department of Health and Human Services, Office of the Assistant Secretary for Planning and Evaluation.

48. Under SSI rules, if families pay a third party for an SSI recipient's private room, the SSI benefit is reduced according to the amount contributed up to a maximum of a third of the benefit. Medicaid rules regarding the effect of family supplementation on Medicaid eligibility are ambiguous, particularly for persons who are not eligible for SSI, because states have the option of disregarding certain income.

49. Mollica, R. (2002). op.cit.

50. No applicable federal statutes exist other than the Keys Amendment to the Social Security Act, which is applicable to board and care facilities in which a "substantial number of SSI recipients" are likely to reside. However, the Keys amendment is virtually unused to address quality. General Accounting Office. (1989) *Board and Care: Insufficient Assurances That Residents' Needs Are Identified and Met.* Washington, D.C.

51. Greene, A.M., Hawes, C., Wood, M., and Woodsong, C. (1997). "How Do Family Members Define Quality in Assisted Living Facilities?" *Generations*, Vol. 21, No. 4, pp. 34-36. Hawes, C. et al. (December 1999). op.cit.

52. United States General Accounting Office. (1999) *Assisted Living: Quality of Care and Consumer Protection Issues in Four States.* GAO/HEHS-99-27.

53. Ibid.

54. Hawes, C., and Phillips, C.D. (2000). *High Services or High Privacy Assisted Living Facilities, Their Residents and Staff: Results from a National Survey.* Office of Disability, Aging, and Long-Term Care Policy, Office of the Assistant Secretary for Planning and Evaluation, U.S. Department of Health and Human Services.

55. Ibid.

56. O'Keeffe, J. et al. (July 2003). op.cit.

57. Goldsteain, A. "Better than a nursing home?" *Time*, August 13, 2001, Vol 158, No. 6; Zahn, M. "Lapses in care lead to deaths, records show: Hundreds of residents are at risk in assisted living centers, where too few staffers struggle to care for sicker people." [Online]. Cited in Kissan, S., Gifford, D.R., Mor, V., and Patry, G. "Recommen-

dations for Admission and Continued Stay Criteria for Assisted Living Facilities."
[Paper submitted for publication.]

58. Mollica, R. (2002). op.cit.

59. Hawes, C., and Phillips, C.D. (1999). A *National Study of Assisted Living for the Frail Elderly: Final Summary Report.* Prepared for the Office of Disability, Aging, and Long-Term Care Policy, Office of the Assistant Secretary for Planning and Evaluation, U.S. Department of Health and Human Services.

60. Mollica, R. (2002). op.cit.

61. Mollica, R. (2002). op.cit.

62. O'Keeffe, J. (December 1996). op.cit.

63. O'Keeffe, J. (December 1996). op.cit.

64. However, a law adopted in 2000 prevents the licensing agency from ordering the removal of any resident, if the resident, his/her family, physician and the facility agree to the continued stay and the facility assures that necessary additional services will be provided.

65. Several states allow waivers for facilities to retain residents who otherwise would not meet the criteria and some states combine two or more approaches. Robert Mollica, personal communication, December, 2003.

Public Policy Initiatives
Addressing Supportive Housing:
The Experience of Connecticut

Nancy W. Sheehan
Claudia E. Oakes

SUMMARY. In the face of an aging population and escalating long-term (LTC) spending, Connecticut's LTC system disproportionately relies on institutional care to provide LTC for elderly and non-elderly individuals. In response, policymakers are attempting to reform the LTC system by increasing the use of home and community-based alternatives and expanding the availability of supportive housing options. *[Article copies available for a fee from The Haworth Document Delivery Service: 1-800-HAWORTH. E-mail address: <docdelivery@haworthpress.com> Website: <http://www.HaworthPress.com> © 2004 by The Haworth Press, Inc. All rights reserved.]*

Nancy W. Sheehan, PhD, and Claudia E. Oakes, MS, OTR/L, are affiliated with the University of Connecticut, and Information Brokering for Long-Term Care, a project of the Center for Home Care Policy & Research of the Visiting Nurse Service of New York.

Information used to develop this case study was obtained from public documents and reports, interviews with federal and state officials, provider organizations, consumer and advocacy groups, and other stakeholders.

Funded by the Robert Wood Johnson Foundation.

[Haworth co-indexing entry note]: "Public Policy Initiatives Addressing Supportive Housing: The Experience of Connecticut." Sheehan, Nancy W., and Claudia E. Oakes. Co-published simultaneously in *Journal of Housing for the Elderly* (The Haworth Press, Inc.) Vol. 18, No. 3/4, 2004, pp. 81-113; and: *Linking Housing and Services for Older Adults: Obstacles, Options, and Opportunities* (eds: Jon Pynoos, Penny Hollander Feldman, and Joann Ahrens) The Haworth Press, Inc., 2004, pp. 81-113. Single or multiple copies of this article are available for a fee from The Haworth Document Delivery Service [1-800- HAWORTH, 9:00 a.m. - 5:00 p.m. (EST). E-mail address: docdelivery@haworthpress.com].

KEYWORDS. Long-term care, housing, aging, affordable, public policy, Connecticut, assisted living

Objectives

This case study examines Connecticut's supportive housing policies and programs in the context of the state's overall efforts to reform LTC. In the past, housing with services was not considered a significant element of the state's LTC system; however, recent efforts to expand community-based supports have resulted in an increasing emphasis on supportive housing as the third tier of LTC, in addition to nursing homes and community-based care.

As policymakers have addressed supportive housing for the elderly, the needs of non-elderly persons with disabilities have also come to the forefront. A growing awareness that many LTC issues transcend the elderly and involve persons of all ages has resulted in increasing attention to supportive housing legislation and initiatives for younger persons with disabilities. The housing initiatives for persons with disabilities have followed different trajectories than those for the elderly for many reasons. They have different advocates, different regulatory demands, and different state agency oversight; however, some convergence has occurred as the scope of LTC has broadened to include persons of all ages. While the primary concern of this case study is Connecticut's supportive housing initiatives for the elderly, information about supportive housing for non-elderly persons is also presented.

Findings

The significant trends that have influenced the expansion of supportive housing in Connecticut are similar to those in most states. These trends include the aging of the population, escalating state expenditures for LTC, and comprehensive LTC planning efforts. *However, at the same time, the pressures on Connecticut are particularly acute because nursing homes have been the major component of the state's LTC system.* Further, the state's per capita spending on LTC is the highest of any state except New York (AARP, 2002).

Housing, particularly supportive housing, is a critical component of the LTC infrastructure. Unlike other states, such as Oregon, which developed extensive community-based residential alternatives dating back to the 1980s, Connecticut has *only recently expanded its thinking about residential alternatives.*

The state's multi-agency housing structure complicates the process of adding services to housing. *The absence of a single agency assuming a leadership role in the development, implementation, and oversight of supportive housing programs when services are added can lead to programs that lack a guiding philosophy or operational framework for how housing and services for frail elders should work together.* No one agency has legitimate authority or responsibility for developing, implementing, and monitoring an overall vision for ensuring the quality of life of elders. Nor is there a single agency or legislative committee that provides oversight for the supportive housing initiative per se. The lack of a lead agency is particularly problematic because of the inherent complexity that arises when housing and supportive services are combined (Kane & Kane, 2002; Schuetz, 2003; Sheehan & Oakes, 2003a).

Supportive Housing Programs for the Elderly

Connecticut's supportive housing programs for the elderly are designed to reduce reliance on nursing homes by delivering services to frail elders who without such assistance would need to relocate to a nursing home. Connecticut's major supportive housing initiatives involve several models of affordable assisted living (AL) developed over the last few years.

1. *Assisted Living Services (ALS) in State-Subsidized Congregate Housing:* All state-subsidized elderly congregate housing facilities are eligible to participate in the ALS program designed to offer services to frail elderly residents who meet the functional eligibility requirements for the state home care program. In addition to receiving the existing service package in CH (weekly housekeeping, one meal per day, social and recreational programming, and 24-hour emergency response), eligible residents may receive assisted living services. Funds for the ALS program come from either the Connecticut Home Care Program for Elders (CHCPE) or a Department of Economic and Community Development (DECD) subsidy providing up to $500 for residents who exceed financial eligibility for the home care program. From the beginning of the program May 2001 to June 30, 2003, a total of 269 residents received ALS.
2. *Assisted Living Services in Federally Subsidized Senior Housing:* Four federally subsidized senior housing complexes were authorized under legislation passed in 2000 and 2001 to provide ALS under the state's Medicaid waiver program. Three complexes are currently operational. Of these, two provide the additional DECD service subsidy for residents who do not qualify for the CHCPE. From May 2001 to June 30, 2003, 150 elderly residents have received ALS. Additionally, in November 2002, Connecticut was one of 12 states that received HUD funds to convert three multifamily housing complexes to provide assisted living. When the conversions are complete, these three complexes should serve a total of approximately 100 elderly residents.
3. *Demonstration Project to Offer 300 Units of Affordable Assisted Living:* Legislation to create 300 units of affordable AL was passed in 1998 and 1999. Responsibility for implementing the program is shared among the

Department of Social Services (DSS), DECD, and Connecticut Housing Finance Authority (CHFA). DSS is responsible for applying for a waiver to secure federal financial participation to fund ALS, establish a process to select providers, and determine the number of dwelling units in the demonstration project. DECD is responsible for the rental assistance program (RAP) or subsidy certificates and CHFA is responsible for the financing of the projects. Of the five planned sites, groundbreaking has occurred at 2 sites, which are expected to be operational in 2004. The remaining three sites are expected to be open in 2005.

4. *Private Assisted Living Pilot Legislation:* Legislation passed in 2002 authorized a pilot program to allow seniors to remain in private assisted living facilities after depleting their assets. This program has two components: (1) a Medicaid waiver for up to 50 people, and (2) a state-funded pilot for 25 elders who qualify for the state funded portion of the home care program. The pilot program pays for the service component but not the rent, so participants may have to obtain family support or negotiate a reduced rate from the facility. Beginning January 1, 2003, 30 elders who live in 13 facilities are participating in this program, and 94 are on the waiting list.

5. *Service Coordination:* Service Coordinators (SC) are employed in a wide range of residential settings (federally subsidized senior housing, state subsidized elderly housing, Congregate Housing Services Program (CHSP), and private and state-subsidized assisted living) in Connecticut. State assisted living regulations mandate the presence of a SC. In addition, DECD provides grants to housing authorities, municipal authorities, and nonprofit corporations operating elderly housing to fund SCs under the Elderly Rental Registry and Counselor Program. Multiple funding sources (DECD, HUD, CHSP, a project's residual receipts) pay for SCs.

6. *Congregate Housing Services Program (CHSP) in Federally Subsidized Housing:* Since the early 1990s, DSS in conjunction with two Area Agencies on Aging (AAAs) has received CHSP grant funding from Rural Housing Services (formerly Farmers' Home Administration) to provide non-medical supportive services to elderly residents in rural elderly housing complexes. Using a "circuit rider" approach, each AAA employs a SC who works with housing complexes in his/her region. A total of 11 sites participate in the program. While the partnership underlying the CHSP is evident in the funding formula (HUD pays 30-40%, the state match from the AAA pays for 50% of expenses, and clients pay from 10 to 20%), financial monitoring of monthly costs is time consuming. Title III funds from the Older Americans Act provide the state match.

Other Supportive Housing Programs

Connecticut's supportive housing initiatives addressing the needs of younger persons with mental illness, chemical dependency, homelessness or risk of homelessness have received recognition for their creative approach involving both capital and subsidy funding to create permanent service-rich housing for low-income persons with disabilities. *These initiatives serve as models for innovative collaborations involving a mix of public and private partnerships, interagency collaborations, and state, federal, or state-federal funding.* Highlights of three innovative programs are presented to gain perspective on the issues around housing initiatives in Connecticut.

1. *Connecticut Supportive Housing Demonstration:* As early as 1993, Connecticut in partnership with the CSH and many state agencies, private philanthropic organizations and foundations, and local providers, established 9 service-enhanced permanent housing complexes (281 total apartments) throughout the state to serve as alternatives to homeless shelters. A comprehensive evaluation of the project provided convincing evidence that the program increased use of support services designed to assist participants in remaining in the community and decreased use of more expensive Medicaid expenses for inpatient care. In addition, the program resulted in improved quality of life among tenants (CSH, 2002).
2. *New Pilots Supportive Housing Initiative:* Based on the success of the CSH demonstration, this initiative is designed to provide a range of permanent supportive housing options throughout the state. This demonstration involves the cooperation of more than 50 public and private agencies to provide 650 individuals with service-enriched housing. In addition to CHFA, which reviews and oversees the proposed projects, other state agencies in the project include DMHAS, DSS, and DECD. Private foundations, local developers and service providers have cooperated to develop an array of housing and services.
3. *CMS Systems Change Grants: Nursing Facilities Transition and Community Integration:* Connecticut is the recipient of two Centers for Medicare and Medicaid Services (CMS) Systems Change grants designed to enable persons with disabilities to live in the least restrictive environment: *Nursing Facilities Transition* and *Community Integration.* These major initiatives are designed to facilitate the integration of persons with disabilities into the community.

Supportive housing initiatives for non-elderly disabled persons reflect a broader range of strategies that emphasize autonomy and inclusion in the community. These include permanent housing for homeless or at-risk persons, which provides an extensive range of services, a program to transition people out of nursing homes, and community-based programs designed to reduce barriers to integration. While the state is beginning to plan for an AL pilot program for individuals with mental retardation, AL is not an option for younger persons with disabilities.

Connecticut's investment in supportive housing reflects the state's dedication to expanding LTC options and choices with the goal of providing care in the least restrictive settings. By expanding options, policymakers hope that reliance on nursing homes will be dramatically reduced. Currently, 52% of Medicaid LTC recipients in Connecticut receive institutional care. Through concerted efforts to expand home- and community-based LTC options, policymakers hope to serve three-quarters of Medicaid LTC clients in the community by 2025. To achieve this goal, there must be a one percent increase every year in Medicaid LTC clients receiving services in the community.

Policy Implications

Connecticut faces issues (e.g., cost-containment, LTC planning, transitioning people out of nursing homes, and community integration) similar to those that are being confronted by most states (Coleman, Fox-Grage, & Folkemer, July 2003). Thus Connecticut's experience in developing supportive housing can provide valuable lessons for other states:

- *Strong, Effective Leadership:* Many of the LTC reforms have been made possible because of strong, effective leadership at a high level in the Executive Branch.
- *Knowledgeable Housing Finance Professionals:* The ability of individuals in the state housing finance agency to develop a financial package for housing has been key to many of the initiatives.
- *Comprehensive LTC Planning:* The establishment of a comprehensive planning committee is important to focus attention on the complexity of the LTC system for all persons with disabilities.
- *Partnerships:* Successful supportive housing initiatives are based on partnerships among many different agencies, service providers, and private organizations, and in some instances, technical assistance and training are necessary to mobilize the necessary financial and service package.
- *Staff Education and Culture Change:* Educational resources are needed to help professionals from different fields come together and develop initiatives outside the boundaries of their traditional domains.

Policymakers are well aware that despite significant improvements in Connecticut's LTC system for the elderly over the past several years (which include elimination of the waiting list for home care, expanded income eligibility for state-funded home care, and affordable AL initiatives), creating a LTC system that promotes real choice for care in the least restrictive environment necessitates a sustained commitment. In the face of budget deficits, Connecticut's investment in supportive housing initiatives for elderly and non-elderly persons with disabilities reflects the state's dedication to expanding choices. However, in most instances, the state's financial investment in supportive housing initiatives for the elderly (affordable AL programs and SC) has occurred without research to document the impact of these initiatives. This is less true for some of the supportive housing initiatives for non-elderly disabled, which have included a research or evaluation component.

The ongoing efforts of the state's LTC Planning Committee have had a profound influence in thinking about LTC issues. As the Committee seeks to reform the LTC system, the scope of its planning efforts has expanded to include disabled persons of all ages and their families.

This case study will enable other states to learn from Connecticut's efforts to develop meaningful supportive housing choices as part of its comprehensive LTC planning process.

INTRODUCTION

As Connecticut moves into the 21st century, one of the biggest challenges facing policymakers is the financing and delivery of LTC services (State of Connecticut, 2001). To meet this challenge, policymakers are attempting to revamp the state's LTC system to create a comprehensive, cost-effective and responsive system that balances nursing home and community-based care. In the effort to curb the growth of Medicaid spending, combining housing with supportive services has emerged as one of the most important aspects of LTC (Connecticut General Assembly Legislative Program Review and Investigation Committee, 1996; State of Connecticut, 2001). This case study details the supportive housing initiatives that Connecticut has funded as part of the state's efforts to reform LTC.

The term "supportive housing" refers to a range of residential approaches designed to meet the needs of at risk populations, such as homeless persons or "poor people who need assistance with LTC but do not need intensive nursing services" (Connecticut General Assembly Legislative Program Review and Investigation Committee, 1996, p. 57). Other terms used to describe this approach include "service-rich," "service-enhanced" or "housing with services." Supportive housing strategies may involve either adding services to existing housing or developing new residential alternatives. The central feature of supportive housing is that it offers affordable, independent living with services. In contrast to more restrictive settings, supportive housing seeks to enhance residents' autonomy.

The Aging Population and Escalating LTC Spending

The significant trends that have influenced the expansion of supportive housing in Connecticut are similar to those in most states. These trends include the aging of the population, escalating state expenditures for LTC, and comprehensive LTC planning efforts. *However, at the same time, the pressures on Connecticut are particularly acute because nursing homes have been the major component of the state's LTC system.* Further, the state's per capita spending on LTC is the highest of any state except New York (AARP, 2002).

Connecticut has identified LTC reform as an urgent public policy issue, in part due to the projected growth of the elderly population (State of Connecticut, 2001):

- Between 1990 and 2000, the population of residents >65 years of age grew 5.4%. During this same period, the oldest-old (>85) increased by 36.8 % (AARP, 2002). (See Chart 1.)
- Currently, 13.8% of the state's population is 65 years of age and over (470,183 persons) and 1.9% is 85 years of age and over (64,273 persons) (U.S. Census Bureau, Census 2000).
- Future projections indicate that by 2020, 17.4% of the state's population will be 65 years of age and over and 2.0% will be 85 years of age and over (AARP, 2002).

Connecticut's expenditures for LTC are higher than almost all other states and have increased dramatically in recent years:

- Connecticut ranks second highest in per capita spending for LTC ($537.70) (AARP, 2002).
- In 2001, state Medicaid expenditures totaled nearly $3.4 billion, with 54.4% of this amount covering long-term care (LTC) (State of Connecticut, 2003).
- In 2003, Connecticut's expenditures for LTC represented 15% of total expenditures for the state (State of Connecticut, 2003).
- From 1990 to 2002, annual state spending for nursing home care increased from $500 million to over 1 billion, an increase of 106.8% (Ryan, 2002b). (See Chart 2.).

Connecticut's LTC system has disproportionately utilized nursing homes: 6.3% of Connecticut's elders reside in a nursing home, compared to 4.5% of all elders in the U.S. Connecticut spends a higher percentage of its health care spending on nursing homes (15%) than any other state (AARP Public Policy Institute, 2002). In comparison to Oregon, a state of similar size and number of elderly, Connecticut has over three times the number of elderly residents in nursing homes (29,116 versus 9,444). In 2001, Connecticut's total LTC spending was $1.8 billion compared to $1.1 billion for Oregon (Connecticut LTC Planning Committee, 12/3/03). Other indicators of Connecticut's institutional bias include:

- Despite a slight decline in the number of nursing home beds (-1.9%) from 1996 to 2000, Connecticut ranks 15th in the ratio of nursing home beds per 1000 persons 65 years of age and over (61/1000) (AARP, 2002).
- In Connecticut, 52% of Medicaid LTC clients receive assistance in institutional settings (NFs, ICF/MRs and chronic disease hospitals), while 48% receive home- and community-based services (home care, adult day care, and AL) (State of Connecticut, 2003).
- State budget projections for FY 2003 indicate 70% of Medicaid LTC expenditures ($1.9 billion) will pay for institutional care. (State of Connecticut, 2003). (See Chart 3.)
- Projections indicate that if the state does not change its current ratio of LTC spending (70% of Medicaid LTC funds for institutional care and 30% for home- and community-based care), long-term costs will increase to almost $6.4 billion in 2025 (State of Connecticut, 2003).

Key State Agencies Involved in LTC and Supportive Services

The Office of Policy and Management (OPM), a high-level executive-branch agency with major budget responsibility, has been the lead agency responsible for coordinating the state's LTC planning efforts. In this role, OPM has been a strong advocate for affordable supportive housing initiatives to rebalance the LTC system. Other state agencies involved in LTC include the Department of Mental Retardation (DMR), Department of Economic and Community Development (DECD), Department of Public Health (DPH), Department of Mental Health and Addiction Services (DMHAS), Office of Health Care Access (OHCA), Department of Social Services (DSS), and Department of Transportation (DOT). These agencies, as a matter of course, administer programs and services for persons who need assistance due to physical frailty, chronic mental illness, substance abuse, developmental disability, cognitive impairments, or some combination of needs. Programs typically target a particular group (elderly or younger persons with disabilities) or need (mental health care, protection and advocacy, housing and/or transportation). *Barriers to receiving services have included conflicting eligibility requirements, lack of knowledge about services, fragmentation or the lack of comprehensive services, and waiting lists* (Sheehan, 1992; Tilson & Fahey, 1990).

CHART 1. Increase in Connecticut Population, by Age Group (1990-2000)

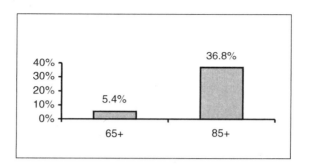

CHART 2. Connecticut Nursing Home Expenditures (in billions)

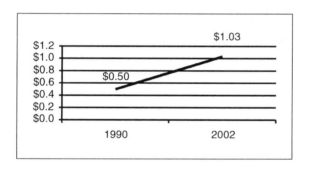

CHART 3. Connecticut's FY 2003 Budgeted Medicaid LTC Spending ($1.9 billion)

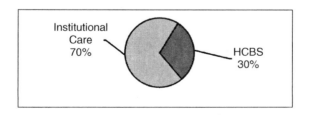

History of the LTC Advisory Group and the LTC Planning Committee

An investigation of Connecticut's home care program conducted in 1996 concluded that the state did not have an adequate LTC system in part because existing programs in three identified component areas (nursing homes, supportive housing, and community-based services) operated with separate and distinct requirements (Connecticut General Assembly Legislative Program Review and Investigation Committee, 1996). A recommendation from this report was the establishment of *an interagency committee "to exchange information on LTC issues, ensure coordinated policy development, and establish a long-term care plan. The plan shall integrate all three major components* of the long-care system" (Connecticut General Assembly Legislative Program Review and Investigation Committee, 1996, pp. 97-98). Since DSS administers many different programs related to LTC (such as home care, rate setting for nursing homes, homes for the aged, home health agencies, Certificates of Need, and Older Americans Act funding), it was given responsibility to develop a plan along with DPH, OHCA, and DECD. (Appendix A presents a glossary of state agencies and programs.)

Subsequently, legislation (PA 98-239) passed in 1998 mandated formation of the LTC Planning Committee and an advisory group, the LTC Advisory Council. They were initially charged with *assessing the LTC needs* of elders and *making recommendations* to ensure an affordable and efficient system that integrates "home care and community-based services, supportive housing arrangements and nursing facilities" (§ 17b-337). Input from public hearings and forums identified several needs related to supportive housing for elders: the need for affordable and accessible supportive housing, supports to encourage aging in place and the need for better reimbursement methods to assist with housing needs (LTC Planning Committee, 1999). The Planning Committee consists of representatives from state agencies involved in LTC and the Chairs and Ranking Members of three legislative committees (Human Services, Public Health, and Aging), while consumers, providers, and advocates compose the Advisory Council.

Since its inception, the committee has been expanded several times. In 1999, DMR, DMHAS, and DOT were added (PA 99-28, 1999), while in 2001, the Department of Children and Families (DCF) and Office of Protection and Advocacy for Persons with Disabilities (P & A) were added to broaden its scope to plan for "all persons in need of long-term care" (PA 01-119, 2001). In addition to expanding both the membership and the mission of the Planning Committee, this act also mandated that *when any LTC program is developed or modified by any state agency, the resulting program must support informal caregivers and consumer-directed choice.* Finally in October 2002, legislation

(PA 02-100) added 8 new members to the LTC Advisory Group. (See Appendix B, which lists the full membership of both groups.)

The Planning Committee also has assumed *oversight for the state's community integration plan to comply with the Supreme Court's Olmstead decision,* which called for community integration for all persons with disabilities. DSS, the lead agency for persons with disabilities, developed the plan "*Choices Are for Everyone: Continuing Toward Community-Based Supports in Connecticut*" (March 2002) based on input from stakeholders and with the advice and assistance from a community task force. The plan proposes four actions steps:

1. *Transition* persons out of nursing homes
2. Expand accessible and affordable *housing options*
3. Expand available *community supports*
4. Facilitate *community connections*

As progress is made toward greater integration, the Planning Committee will regularly review and update the plan.

Connecticut's evolving LTC framework is presented in the Planning Committee's reports (1999 and 2001) and the 2004 draft plan. As amended (PA 01-119, 2001), reports must be submitted every three years to the Human Services and Public Health committees and Select Committee on Aging. The focus of the most recent LTC plan, *"Balancing the system: Working toward real choice for LTC in Connecticut,"* calls for a balancing of the ratio of institutional and home- and community-based care and balancing public and private resources. Recommendations involving supportive housing include:

* Creating *incentives for nursing facilities to convert* to AL or independent living facilities that emphasize consumer direction and choice
* Expanding AL options for *non-elderly* persons
* Increasing utilization of Section 8 *vouchers* so additional vouchers may be requested from HUD
* Establishing a Resident Services *Coordinator in every state-funded elderly housing complex* (State of Connecticut, 2003)

SUPPORTIVE HOUSING IN THE LTC SYSTEM

Housing, particularly supportive housing, is a critical component of the LTC infrastructure. Unlike other states, such as Oregon, which developed extensive community-based residential alternatives dating back to the 1980s,

Connecticut has *only recently expanded its thinking about residential alternatives*. For the state, 1996 stands out as a watershed year. In that year, recommendations from an investigation of state home care program and passage of PA 96-245 which established the Congregate Housing Task Force to study and make recommendations about state-subsidized elderly congregate housing (CH) led to a series of legislative and policy changes intended to radically alter the existing LTC system for elders and expand supportive housing options. The sequence and timing of events for policy reform is outlined in Table 1.

In addition, as Connecticut attempts to comply with the Olmstead decision, there is increased attention on ways that supportive housing can be used to ensure that *all persons with disabilities* (for example, developmental disabilities, chronic mental illness and chemical dependency) can receive care in the least restrictive environments. However, despite efforts to develop a comprehensive LTC approach, *most supportive housing programs in Connecticut still serve different groups* (elderly, developmentally disabled, mentally retarded, and/or mentally ill), are *managed by different agencies*, have *different stakeholders*, and have *different eligibility requirements*. As previously noted, this case study primarily focuses on supportive housing for older persons, but the non-elderly are referred to because of the expanded scope of the LTC Planning Committee.

Connecticut's State Housing Agencies

Unlike some states with a single housing agency, Connecticut relies on *three agencies* to address affordable housing issues. Consequently, housing

TABLE 1. Timeline for Connecticut Policy Reform

Date	Policy Reform
1996	Legislative Program Review & Investigation Committee Report on the state home care program
1997	Congregate Housing Task Force Report
January 1997	No waiting list policy for the state home care program for elders
January 1998	Waiting list for home care program eliminated
July 1998	Authorization of pilot program to offer AL services in a state-funded congregate housing
1998	Legislation authorizing Demonstration project to build 300 units of affordable AL
January 2001	AL services authorized for all state congregate housing sites and two HUD pilot AL programs
January 2003	Private AL pilot legislation

initiatives rely on partnerships among a number of state agencies. The responsibilities for the three agencies are described below:

- *Connecticut Housing Finance Authority (CHFA)*–The state housing finance agency determines the "mix" of *capital funding* (bond financing, federal tax credits, etc.) necessary for creating supportive housing units.
- *Department of Economic and Community Development (DECD)*–The community development agency oversees the *distribution of funds* from U.S. Department of Housing and Urban Development (HUD), including the HOME program and Community Development Block Grant (CDBG) funds and develops the state's overall housing *agenda*. DECD also provides *rental assistance* for elders, funding *for Service Coordinators*, and oversees the ALS program in state-funded congregate housing.
- *Department of Social Services (DSS)*–The primary human service agency provides funding for ALS through its *state and Medicaid waiver home care program* (CHCPE–Connecticut Home Care Program for Elders) and administers the state rental assistance program and Section 8 Voucher programs (including the Section 8 Mainstream Housing Opportunities Program for Persons with Disabilities and the Nursing Facility Transition Preference Program that enables persons with disabilities to live independently in the community).

The state's multi-agency housing structure complicates the process of adding services to housing. *The absence of a single agency assuming a leadership role in the development, implementation, and oversight of supportive housing programs when services are added can lead to programs that lack a guiding philosophy or operational framework for how housing and services for frail elders should work together.* No one agency has legitimate authority or responsibility for developing, implementing, and monitoring an overall vision for ensuring the quality of life of elders. Nor is there a single agency or legislative committee that provides oversight for the supportive housing initiative per se. The lack of a lead agency is particularly problematic because of the inherent complexity that arises when housing and supportive services are combined (Kane & Kane, 2002; Schuetz, 2003; Sheehan & Oakes, 2003a).

Recognizing the Unmet Needs of Elderly and Non-Elderly Persons with Disabilities

Connecticut policymakers increasingly acknowledge that inattention to the needs of vulnerable or at-risk elderly and disabled persons ultimately results in higher budgetary expenditures. Costs accrued when needs are not met include expensive institutional care, emergency room care, inpatient medical and psychiatric care, and emergency shelter costs. As advocates have argued, Connecticut can no longer afford to ignore the supportive housing needs of persons with disabilities.

Over the last 20 years, elderly residents in subsidized housing have become an increasingly vulnerable group at risk for nursing home placement. The increased prevalence of elderly residents with cognitive and physical impairments has resulted in growing numbers of elders with unmet needs. Since elderly residents in subsidized housing possess multiple factors for nursing home placement (including advanced age, female, poor, living alone, more health problems, more hospitalizations, and smaller support networks) (Black, Rabins, German, McGuire, & Roca, 1997; Morris, Gutkin, Ruchlin & Sherwood, 1990; Rabins, Black, German, Roca, McGuire, Brant & Cook, 1996; Schlesinger & Morris, 1982), supportive housing interventions to meet their needs may prevent or forestall relocation to nursing homes. Although concerns about the unmet needs of elderly residents in Connecticut were expressed as early as the mid-1980s (Sheehan & Mahoney, 1984), programmatic responses to address these needs were slow to develop.

Estimating the numbers and needs of non-elderly persons with disabilities is a daunting task since they do not represent any single categorical group. Younger persons with disabilities include people with developmental disabilities, mental retardation, mental illness, substance abuse, and AIDS. Most estimates concerning the numbers of non-elderly persons with disabilities in Connecticut come from a number of different sources. Using data from the 2002 Current Population Survey, 5.5% of non-institutionalized Connecticut adults in the 18-64 year age range report some disability (n = 114,000) (Houtenville, 2003). DECD has prioritized housing for special needs populations in the state because *as a group they experience a major risk for homelessness.* DECD estimates that a disabled person receiving SSI in Connecticut must pay 84% of his/her monthly income for a one-bedroom apartment. Therefore, a major emphasis of state housing policy is to develop affordable accessible housing for disabled persons who are either homeless or near homeless.

EXPANSION OF COMMUNITY-BASED OPTIONS

Connecticut's LTC reform efforts to expand community-based options for elders, particularly its affordable AL models, have received national recognition. In all, the state has pursued six sets of initiatives:

1. ALS in state-subsidized CH
2. ALS in federally subsidized senior housing
3. ALS in private pay facilities

4. Development of purpose-built affordable AL settings
5. Service Coordination (SC) across a range of federally and state-subsidized buildings
6. CHSP

By September 2004, Connecticut expects that up to 600 low- and moderate-income elders will be receiving ALS under all AL initiatives (*www.dss.state.ct.us/presssel/092903.htm*).

Funding and Regulation of the ALS Component

The service component of the state's affordable housing options is funded through the Connecticut Home Care Program for Elders (CHCPE) under either the Medicaid Waiver or state portion of the program, which is administered by DSS. Additionally, in state-funded CH facilities and two federally funded elderly housing complexes DECD provides a subsidy of up to $500 for residents who do not financially qualify for CHCPE. No funding is provided for the housing component.

The Department of Public Health (DPH) has played a significant role in the development of affordable AL options. State regulations mandate that *DPH must license the agency* that provides ALS (an Assisted Living Services Agency or ALSA) and *regulate the residential setting* (Managed Residential Community or MRC). According to regulations, the MRC *settings* should provide three meals per day, laundry service, transportation, housekeeping, chore services, recreational and social programming, an on-site service coordinator, 24-hour security, emergency call systems, and a common area (Regulation 19-13-D105 (a) 13).

Regulations governing the ALSA include a nurse on-site 20 hours each week. However, the Commissioner of Public Health has waived some of these regulations (such as three meals per day and laundry service) in order to deliver ALS to frail elderly residents in subsidized housing settings (federally-subsidized senior housing and state-subsidized CH). The 20-hour on-site nursing requirement was also reduced. *Flexibility in waiving some regulations makes it possible to offer the ALS program in congregate and senior housing settings.*

In accordance with state regulations, ALS are provided by a licensed ALSA, which may be a unit in a home health care agency. The ALSA provides limited nursing and personal care and instrumental support (such as housekeeping, laundry, meal preparation), as specified in individual care plans for each resident. Services are delivered in residential settings ranging from federally subsidized senior housing to private AL facilities. (See Table 2 for a summary of the four AL packages.)

TABLE 2. Summary of AL Packages

Level	Hours Per Week	Billable Daily Charge
1	1 - 3	$16.32
2	4 - 8	$31.88
3	9 - 15	$47.53
4	15 - 25	$66.30

The program is flexible to accommodate changes in residents' needs (e.g., discharge from hospital) so that the level of the service package may change during the course of a month. Payment for ALS for each client is calculated based on the total billing days at each level for the month. Program statistics for October 2003 for each of the different housing settings (congregates, HUD complexes, and private AL) are presented in Appendix C. While the totals vary as a function of the number of participants, the figures suggest differences across settings in the relative distribution of the service levels.

Assisted Living Services in State-Subsidized Congregate Housing

State-subsidized CH serves frail elderly (62 years of age and over) with incomes up to 80% of the area median. Elderly applicants to CH must need assistance with one or more activities of daily living. Residents of CH live in private apartments. The service package consists of weekly housekeeping, one meal per day, social and recreational programming, and 24-hour emergency response.

Based on the success of a 12-month state-funded pilot program ($100,000) designed to bring ALS to a subset of residents in a single congregate facility (Sheehan, 1999), the General Assembly authorized a program to allow ALS in all state-funded elderly CH (PA 00-2, June Special Session, CGS 8-119m, 17b-342c). The program permits the CHCPE to pay for services for those who qualify and DECD to pay for some residents who do not qualify financially. Three agencies (DSS, DECD, and DPH) were mandated to implement the program in state-funded CH facilities that agreed to participate in the program. Each agency was responsible for a different facet of the program:

- State-funded CH was represented by DECD
- DPH covered licensure and oversight of the ALSA
- DSS determined eligibility and funding under the Medicaid waiver (Medicaid and state-funded portion) to pay for services

DECD, DPH, and DSS shared responsibility for developing policies and procedures for determining eligibility, specifying the procedures for accessing services, and modifying regulations concerning the ALSA and MRC appropriate to the different settings. An investigation of CH directors' perceptions of the ALS program in their facilities revealed *confusion about the policies and procedures governing the delivery of the services* (for example, admission policies, privacy of information between the MRC and ALSA). Further, the directors' descriptions of the *features of the ALS program* in their housing (availability of nurse on-site, eligibility to receive services, communication between housing and ALS staff, issues of confidentiality and privacy, and overall frailty levels among participants) *varied widely across sites* (Sheehan & Oakes, 2003b).

Sixteen of the 24 state-subsidized congregates participate in the program. Residents who are already receiving services from CHCPE have the right to refuse ALS and continue to receive fee-for-service home care services. From the beginning of the program May 2001 to June 30, 2003, a total of 269 residents received ALS. The number of active AL participants in state-funded CH as of October 31, 2003 was 166. Of these, 28 are under Medicaid, 49 under the state-funded home care program, and 89 receive a DECD subsidy.

Assisted Living Services in Federally Subsidized Senior Housing

Most AL programs in federally subsidized senior housing in Connecticut involve a *partnership between the state and federal governments*. Four federally subsidized senior housing complexes in the state were authorized under legislation passed in 2000 and 2001 (PA 00-2, JSS and PA 01-2, JSS, CGS 8-206e (d)) to provide ALS under the state's Medicaid waiver program. While up to four housing complexes may participate, only three complexes are currently operating under this program. Only two of these three sites provide the DECD service subsidy for residents who do not qualify for the CHCPE. From May 2001 to June 30, 2003, 150 elderly residents have received ALS. There are currently 106 residents receiving ALS in all three complexes. Of these, 25 are funded by Medicaid, 29 under the state home care program, and 52 through the DECD subsidy.

Connecticut was also one of 12 states in November 2002 that received HUD funds to convert three multifamily housing complexes into AL facilities ($9,774,895). Two of these complexes, at the time of the award, had already been providing ALS for some time. Twelve months after the HUD grants were announced, only two of the three complexes have finalized the paperwork for these conversions. When the conversions are complete, these three complexes should serve a total of approximately 100 elderly residents.

Demonstration Project to Offer 300 Units of Affordable Assisted Living

Legislation in 1998 and 1999 (PA 98-239, PA 99-279, CGS 17b-347e) authorized the Assisted Living Demonstration Project to create 300 units of affordable AL for moderate- and low-income elders. The legislation required DSS, DECD, and CHFA to enter into a Memorandum of Understanding no later than January 1, 1999, which specifies that:

1. DSS apply for a waiver to secure federal financial participation to fund ALS, establish a process to select providers, and determine the number of dwelling units in the demonstration project;
2. DECD provide the rental assistance program (RAP) or subsidy certificates; and,
3. CHFA provide second mortgage loans for housing projects for which the authority has provided financial assistance in the form of a loan secured by a first mortgage pursuant to section 8-403 of the general statutes for the demonstration project.

CHFA issued a request for proposals to participate in the demonstration project by July 1, 1999 with June 8, 2001 as a deadline for applications. However, significant *delays plagued the early stages* of the project. Therefore, a new RFP (PA 01-2, JSS, § 37) was issued for proposals on July 1, 2001. While the final report for this demonstration was due on January 1, 2003, groundbreaking for two of the five demonstration sites just occurred in 2003. Two sites are expected to be operational by March and September 2004, respectively. Two are expected in March 2005 and one in September 2005.

Private Assisted Living Pilot Legislation

Legislation passed in 2002 (PA 02-7, May 9 Special Session, CGS 17b-365 & 17b-366) authorized DSS to start two new pilot programs to pay for services in private AL facilities:

- Medicaid waiver pilot for up to 50 people
- State-funded pilot (Sec. 17b-365) for 25 elders whose assets and income qualify them for the state-funded portion of CHCPE

Beginning January 1, 2003, the pilot programs were available to residents in private AL facilities. Eligible individuals must qualify for the CHCPE taking into consideration the Medicaid asset transfer rules. Since the pilot program only pays for the service component, if the resident is unable to pay for room and board, he/she may have to obtain family support or negotiate a reduced rate from the MRC. The ALSA must enroll as a CHCPE provider and accept the ALS rates set by DSS in order to participate in this program. Currently, 13 ALSAs and 35 sites are eligible to participate. There are 30 elders participating in this program who are living in 13 different private AL facilities. Of these, 8 elders are qualified under the Medicaid waiver and 22 elders are under the state home care program. In addition, 94 residents are on a waiting list for the pilot. Twenty-four of these residents are in the process of being screened. The remaining 70 are placed in the "hold" category because they are ineligible due to their functional or financial status or their ALSA or MRC is not participating in the pilot program. After two years, OPM will *evaluate the cost-effectiveness of the pilot program* (Personal communication with DSS staff). A preliminary analysis conducted by the Office of Fiscal Analysis indicates that the expected savings from these two pilot programs is $249,000 (State of Connecticut, 2002). The savings calculation is based on the savings by delaying relocation to a nursing home. The average annual cost of a nursing home stay in Connecticut is approximately $96,000.

Service Coordination

While Service Coordination (SC) emerged in the early 1990s as a strategy to address the needs of frail elderly residents who were aging in place in senior housing, now all AL programs are mandated by the state to employ a service coordinator. Connecticut was among the first states to develop a SC program in the early 1990s (Sheehan, 1993). The model, funded by the Administration on Aging, involved a partnership among CHFA, three private management companies, and the University of Connecticut. According to current Connecticut statute, the role of the service coordinator is to assess residents' needs, assist residents to maintain independence, monitor the delivery of services, maintain regular contact, provide mediation and conflict resolution, and advocate for services.

Currently, service coordinators are employed in a variety of residential settings (federally subsidized senior housing, state elderly housing, CHSP housing sites, CH, and AL facilities). Since different programs and multiple funding sources pay for service coordinators (e.g., DECD, HUD, CHSP, a project's residual receipts), the prevalence of service coordinators in different types of housing is difficult to pinpoint.

DECD provides grants to housing authorities, municipal authorities, and nonprofit corporations operating elderly housing to fund SC under the Elderly Rental Registry and Counselor Program. Proposals for funding must include demonstrated need and matching funds (PA 98-263, HB. 5650). Although funding totaled $800,000 for SC grants in 2002-2003, only $386,000 was awarded. The statute also specifies that a service coordinator should not be responsible for more than 150 units of elderly housing.

Both the state's most recent LTC plan (State of Connecticut, 2003) and the State Plan on Aging highlight the importance of SC for addressing elders' LTC needs. Both plans include goals to increase the presence of service coordinators in elderly housing. The LTC plan due out in 2004 *recommends SC in every state-funded elderly housing complex*. Currently, estimates indicate that only one of three state elderly housing complexes employs a service coordinator (State of Connecticut, 2003).

Congregate Housing Services Program (CHSP) in Federally Subsidized Housing

The CHSP is designed to provide supportive services to residents of federally-subsidized senior housing. With funding from the federal government (HUD or Rural Housing Services), elderly residents and younger persons with disabilities in designated complexes who have at least three ADL or IADL impairments are eligible for services to enable them to remain independent. The CHSP services are non-medical and include housekeeping, personal care, meals, transportation, and other non-medical support. Service coordinators work with residents to develop individualized service plans. A volunteer Professional Assessment Committee (PAC) assists in determining eligibility and reassessing needs.

Since the early 1990s, DSS in conjunction with two Area Agencies on Aging (AAAs) has received CHSP grant funding from Rural Housing Services (formerly Farmers' Home Administration) to provide services in rural elderly housing complexes in two regions in the state. Although most CHSP funded projects are project-based, Connecticut uses a "circuit rider" approach with a service coordinator in each AAA working with participating rural elderly housing complexes in his/her region. The Eastern AAA serves 7 sites, while the Western AAA serves 4 sites. To illustrate the scope of this program, during the past fiscal year, the eastern region's program has served a total of 96 residents in 7 complexes with an active caseload of 79 residents (Personal communication with DSS staff). While the partnership underlying the CHSP is evident in the funding formula (HUD pays 30-40%, the state match from the AAA pays for 50% of expenses, and clients pay from 10 to 20%), financial monitoring of monthly costs is time consuming. Title III funds from the Older Americans Act provide the state match.

SUPPORTIVE HOUSING INITIATIVES FOR THE NON-ELDERLY

Connecticut's supportive housing initiatives addressing the needs of younger persons with mental illness, chemical dependency, homelessness or risk of homelessness have received recognition for their creative approach involving both capital and subsidy funding to create permanent service-rich housing for low-income persons with disabilities. *These initiatives serve as models for innovative collaborations involving a mix of public and private partnerships, interagency collaborations, and state, federal, or state-federal funding.* Highlights of three innovative programs are presented to gain perspective on the issues around housing initiatives in Connecticut.

Connecticut Supportive Housing Demonstration

As early as 1993, Connecticut in partnership with the CSH and many state agencies, private philanthropic organizations and foundations, and local providers, established 9 service-enhanced permanent housing complexes (281 total apartments) throughout the state to serve as alternatives to homeless shelters. Two independent consultant groups conducted a comprehensive evaluation of the demonstration project that involved tracing changes over time in tenants, service utilization, health care costs, and the financial stability of the complexes (Arthur Anderson, LLP, University of Pennsylvania Health System, Department of Psychiatry Center for Mental Health Policy and Services Research, Sherwood, K. E., & TWR Consulting, 2001). Results from the evaluation provided convincing evidence that *supportive housing increased use of support services designed to assist participants in remaining in the community and decreased use of more expensive Medicaid expenses for inpatient care.* For Medicaid-eligible tenants who remained in the housing for three years (n = 126), there was a 71% decrease in average Medicaid reimbursement per tenant for inpatient healthcare. In addition, the program resulted in improved quality of life among tenants (Corporation for Supportive Housing, 2002).

New Pilots Supportive Housing Initiative

The overwhelming success of the CSH demonstration project led to authorization of a New Pilots Supportive Housing Initiative in 1998. This initiative is designed to develop a range of supportive housing options across the state. The program aims to provide housing that is affordable, good quality, safe, and with access to public transportation. This demonstration involves the cooperation of more than 50 public and private agencies to provide 650 individuals with service-enriched housing. In addition to CHFA, which reviews and oversees the proposed projects, other state agencies in the project include DMHAS, DSS, and DECD. Private foundations, local developers and service providers have cooperated to develop an array of housing and services.

Housing units may come from new construction, rehabilitation, acquisition, or leasing of scattered sites. Case management is considered to be the key to providing for individualized needs. Services include: independent living skills training, employment training, peer supports and linkages with other community services. In 2000, during Phase I of the Pilots Program, Connecticut allocated $2.1 million for services through DHMAS. With these funds, DHMAS funded 50 service providers. For several projects, the funding for services provided by the state served as a match to secure rental subsidies through the HUD Continuum of Care Program. Since Phase I was successful, in 2001 Connecticut allocated an additional $3 million for service subsidies to address the support needs of 570 people. In addition, Connecticut has set aside a $23 million financing package (e.g., Low-Income Housing Tax Credits) to fund either the construction of new units or rehabilitation of existing units to create up to 300 new units of additional supportive housing. And most recently, in 2003, $6 million was added to the DMHAS and the CHFA budgets to cover the expenses of expanding the program to support 650 residents.

CMS Systems Change Grants:
Nursing Facilities Transition and Community Integration

Connecticut is the recipient of two Centers for Medicare and Medicaid Services (CMS) Systems Change grants designed to enable persons with disabilities to live in the least restrictive environment: *Nursing Facilities Transition and Community Integration.* These major initiatives are designed to facilitate the integration of persons with disabilities into the community.

In 2001, Connecticut received a three-year, $800,000 grant to facilitate the transition of 150 nursing home residents into the community. The plan includes strong partnerships between numerous state agencies and private partners. The Connecticut Association of Centers for Independent Living (CIL) is responsible for carrying out the project's major activities. A major role of the CILs is to provide training to professionals and nursing home residents who desire to return to the community. The activities include:

- Creating a best practices model for transitions
- Implementing an outreach campaign to educate professionals, persons with disabilities and family members about successful transitions

- Providing training materials regarding independent living to professionals throughout the state
- Recruiting volunteers to provide peer support to persons going through the transition

Information is available from both a toll-free number for anyone interested in exploring independent living options and a guide concerning how to plan the transition. The CILs throughout the state will provide *training in both independent living skills and the philosophy of independent living.* In addition, a "Common Sense Fund" pays for *transitioning costs* not covered by other programs. DSS helps to identify potential residents and the Ombudsman Program disseminates information to residents and their families. DSS has prioritized 40 rental vouchers for transitioning individuals. To date, a total of 40 successful transitions have occurred. A key component of the project is a *comparative cost-benefit analysis* comparing nursing home and community-based care.

In 2002, Connecticut received a three-year, $1.35 million grant through the Real Change Systems Grant to enhance opportunities for independent living for people with disabilities, and to assist three communities to become models of inclusion for people with disabilities. Administrative leadership for the grant is shared between OPM and the University of Connecticut A. J. Pappanikou Center for Excellence. The funded project involves a multi-pronged approach to achieving community inclusion. Activities include developing and conducting a statewide survey of persons with disabilities concerning issues of inclusion, expanding the workforce to provide support, reviewing the training and capacity of state agencies to address the needs of persons with disabilities, and increasing public awareness.

Three cities were awarded Model Community grants to develop programs that will bring about community level changes with the assistance of community-based task forces in each city (Bruder, 2003). Each of the communities selected has its own set of plans/activities designed to promote community inclusion. Targeted goals include improving access to public accommodations, providing sensitivity training to town employees and maximizing employment opportunities for people with disabilities. While none of these initiatives focus directly on housing, they address the broader changes that are necessary for increasing the inclusion of persons with disabilities in the community.

EVALUATING SUPPORTIVE HOUSING INITIATIVES

Given the state's significant investment in developing affordable AL options, systematic research is needed to explore how these services are implemented in different settings and how they impact elders. While some systematic evaluations are underway (e.g., the Nursing Facilities Transition grant, Community Integration project), there is little research to assist policymakers in reaching evidence-based decisions. The variation among different models and residential settings challenges researchers to address how the type of setting, the level of services, and the level of resident need interact to yield different resident outcomes. Research is also needed to assess how different program features impact resident outcomes (e.g., nurse-directed wellness program, health program, or enriched socialization). Further, since residents vary considerably in levels of need and housing managers vary in their tolerance for accommodating physical frailty and cognitive impairment, research is needed to describe how receiving services impacts different subgroups of residents in different settings. Although policymakers have focused primarily on the goal of reducing LTC expenditures, the success of the programs cannot be simply measured in terms of cost savings. AL options must also be researched concerning their impact on quality of life. Clearly, both qualitative and quantitative assessments are necessary to aid policymakers in their decision-making.

Although policymakers have endorsed supportive housing options, particularly AL options as a major LTC cost savings strategy, the lack of any comparative data, quasi-experimental designs, or longitudinal data, limits such conclusions. *What is needed is a comprehensive evaluation of all AL programs, similar to the evaluation of the CSH Supportive Housing Demonstration project, to demonstrate whether these programs reduce Medicaid expenses, improve health or functioning, or enhance quality of life.*

Data for Cost-Benefit Analyses

Policymakers argue that since AL is less expensive than nursing home care it de facto saves money. However, demonstrating cost savings from supportive housing initiatives rests on the ability to prove that the services actually delayed or forestalled relocation to a nursing home, or hospitalization, and in some instances the patchwork of funding and program eligibility requirements impedes the realization of cost savings. Moreover, any effort to determine the cost effectiveness of the services, even for residents receiving the lowest level of services, should factor into the equation the costs to both the resident and his/her family if the services are not provided. Consequently, a more systematic analysis of how level of need impacts service utilization and cost savings is needed.

Impact on Quality of Life

Supportive housing, while serving as an alternative to nursing home care, should enhance the quality of life of persons with disabilities. While state regulations for AL mandate quality assurance procedures (e.g., chart review, review of care plans, patient bill of rights, Professional Assessment Committee, satisfaction surveys, etc.) that are overseen by DPH, these regulations do not adequately address residents' quality of life. Satisfaction surveys may be an unreliable indicator of residents' quality of life because residents are reluctant to complain about the quality of the program lest they be relocated to a nursing home (Sheehan & Oakes, 2003a). Although budgetary constraints may limit more extensive oversight, the variations both within and across the models of AL (e.g., hours of weekly on-site nursing service, core MRC services) and levels of frailty among participants suggest the need for additional oversight to ensure quality of care. Connecticut, unlike other states, has not placed AL under the jurisdiction of the Ombudsman's Office. However, the most recent LTC plan (State of Connecticut, 2003) recommends that the LTC Ombudsman's Office oversee AL facilities as a way of ensuring quality of care and quality of life.

OUTSTANDING POLICY ISSUES

As housing and home care are combined, previous distinctions are becoming blurred, posing new challenges and questions for policymakers (Redfoot & Pandya, 2002). These include:

Regulatory Issues:

- When ALS are added to congregate or federally subsidized senior housing, what are the consequences of *waiving regulations* for the health and well-being of residents?
- As the government is involved in offering ALS, how are the interests of *protecting the resident* and *enhancing autonomy* balanced?
- Is there is an *upper limit of disability* or need for residents in these different residential settings beyond which nursing home care is necessary (Golant, 2003)?
- What is the *appropriate mix of regulatory controls* to ensure quality of care and quality of life in these settings (Golant, 2003)?

Collaboration or Partnerships:

- Since DSS, DECD, and DHP are involved in most affordable AL settings, how can their different ways of viewing residents (home care client, congregate housing resident, and patient) be integrated into *a single, unified model*?
- Given the strong influence of the state home care program on newer models of affordable AL, how can AL programs be *distinguished from traditional home care*?
- Should maximum participation by housing sponsors in supportive housing programs (e.g., ALS programs, SC programs) be encouraged through the *use of incentives*?
- How can federal and state programs (e.g., HUD Assisted Living Conversion grants and ALS programs) be *coordinated* in a more timely fashion?

Integration:

- When services are added to subsidized housing, how can the *residential nature of the housing be maintained*?
- How can *funding streams* to pay for ALS (Medicaid, state home care, and DECD) *be coordinated* to maximize participation and minimize paperwork and confusion among residents?
- Since housing and services are unbundled, what happens *when there are no provisions to cover housing costs* (e.g., when a resident in private AL qualifies for AL services but cannot pay the residential costs)?
- How can incremental changes in addressing LTC for elderly and non-elderly disabled bring about *sufficient systemic change* to alter Connecticut's LTC system?

Level of Service:

- What is the *optimum level of nursing supervision* to ensure quality of care (Hyde, 2001)?
- How does the presence of extremely disabled residents impact the *quality of life of other residents* (Golant, 2003)?

Targeting Services:

- Should services be *targeted to the most needy* elders?

Housing Stock:

- If the strategy only involves adding services to existing housing, how does this address the problem if the state's *supply of affordable housing* is inadequate?

VALUABLE LESSONS FOR OTHER STATES

Connecticut faces issues (e.g., cost-containment, LTC planning, transitioning people out of nursing homes, and community integration) similar to those that are being confronted by most states (Coleman, Fox-Grage, & Folkemer, 2003). Thus Connecticut's experience in developing supportive housing can provide valuable lessons for other states:

1. *Strong, Effective Leadership:* Many of the LTC reforms have been made possible because of the strong, effective leadership of several key individuals in OPM who have provided energetic direction for rebalancing the LTC system. OPM's role has been key because of its elevated position in the Executive Branch and its impact on the highest level budgetary planning.
2. *Knowledgeable Housing Finance Professionals:* Many of the supportive housing initiatives involved in expanding the stock of affordable housing for persons with disabilities have been made possible because of the ability of key individuals in the state housing finance agency to develop a financial package for the housing.
3. *Comprehensive LTC Planning:* The establishment of the LTC Planning Committee has helped to focus attention on the complexity of the LTC system for all persons with disabilities. The current report released by the Planning Committee, which is the first to address the needs of all persons with disabilities, represents the first major step in developing a sufficiently comprehensive plan addressing the needs of all persons with disabilities that goes beyond meeting the needs of only the elderly.
4. *Partnerships:* Successful supportive housing initiatives are based on partnerships among many different agencies, service providers, and private organizations. In some instances, the local providers and service agencies interested in developing supportive housing may need technical assistance and training to mobilize the necessary financial and service package to create housing. It is important to understand why some sponsors of housing for the elderly eligible to participate in AL programs are not interested.
5. *Staff Education and Culture Change:* As new initiatives bring together housing, health care and service professionals, educational resources need to be directed to help professionals understand the overall philosophy of the program, develop policies and procedures, and maintain standards. As professionals from different fields come together to create supportive housing, education should help them think outside the boundaries of the immediate domains to create programs that are centered on individual needs.

In conclusion, as policymakers pursue the challenge of creating supportive housing options for persons with disabilities, they must focus their efforts on creating residential options that maximize individuals' capacity and promote and enhance quality of life (emotional well-being, interpersonal relationships, personal development, physical well-being, self-determination, social inclusion, and rights) (Schalock, DeVries & Lebsack, 1999).

REFERENCES

AARP (2002). *Survey on Assisted Living in Connecticut.* Retrieved November 1, 2003 from: *http://www.org/aarp.org/ct/Articles/a2002-06-26-ct-aliving.html*

Arthur Anderson, LLP, University of Pennsylvania Health System, Department of Psychiatry Center for Mental Health Policy and Services Research, Sherwood, K. E., & TWR Consulting. (2001) *2002 Connecticut Supportive Housing Demonstration Program Evaluation Report.* New Haven, CT: Commissioned by CSH.

Black, B., Rabins, P., German, P., McGuire, M., & Roca, R. (1997). Need and unmet need for mental health care among elderly public housing residents. *The Gerontologist, 37,* 717-728.

Bruder, M.B. (2003 June). Real Choice Systems Change Grant (#P-911541/1). Third Quarterly Report. Farmington, CT: University of Connecticut Health Center: A.J. Pappanikou Center for Excellence in Developmental Disabilities Education, Research, and Service.

Coleman, B., Fox-Grage, W., & Folkemer, D. (2003, July). State long-term care: Recent developments and policy directions: 2003 Policy update. Forum for State Health Policy Leadership, National Conference of State Legislatures. (Produced under HHS/ASPE Contract No. 100-97-0015, D.O. #17).

Coleman, B. (1998). *New directions for state long-term care systems* (2nd ed.). Washington, DC: AARP Public Policy Institute.

Connecticut General Assembly Legislative Program Review & Investigation Committee (1996, December). *Services to the elderly to support daily living.* Hartford, CT.

Cooper, E., & O'Hara, A. (2003, September). *State housing agencies–How they can help people with disabilities.* Opening Doors: A House Publication for the disability community: Technical Assistance Collaborative, Inc. and the Consortium for Citizens with Disabilities Housing Task Force (Issue No. 22). Retrieved November 12, 2003, from: *http://www.c-c-d.org/od-Sept03.htm*

Corporation for Supportive Housing (2002, May). *Connecticut Supportive Housing Demonstration Program: Program Evaluation Final Report* (May 2002). New Haven: Author.

Council of State Governments (2003). *America's Best Innovations: 2003 Innovations Program Winners and Alternates.* Retrieved November 12, 2003, from: *http://www. csg.org/CSG/Programs/innovations/2003+program+winners.htm*

Department of Economic and Community Development. (2002) *2002 Tenant Demographic Report–State of Connecticut.* Retrieved November 12, 2003, from: *http://www. ct.gov/ecd/cwp.view.asp?A=1105&Q=250604*

General Statutes of Connecticut (2003, January 1). (Rev.). Retrieved November 12, 2003 from: *http://www.cga.state.ct.us/2003/pub/Titles.htm*

Golant, S.M. (November 2003). Presentation at the Pre-Conference Workshop, *Assisted Living Research, Policy and Practice: the Status and Future of Translational Research*. Annual Meeting of the Gerontological Society, San Diego, CA.

Gregory, S.R., & Gibson, M.J. (2002). *Across the States 2002: Profiles of Long-Term Care, Connecticut*. Washington, DC: Public Policy Institute, AARP. Retrieved November 12, 2003, from: *http://research.aarp.org/health/d17794_2002_ats_ct.pdf*

Houtenville, A.J. (2003, May 15). *Disability Statistics in the United States*. Ithaca, NY: Cornell University Rehabilitation Research and Training Center, Retrieved November 12, 2003, from: *www.disabilitystatistics.org*.

Hyde, J. (2001). Understanding the context of assisted living. In K.H. Namazi & P.K. Chaftez (Eds.), *Assisted Living: Current Issues in Facility Management and Resident Care* (pp. 15-28). Westport, CT: Auburn House.

Kane, R.L. & Kane, R.A. (2002, November). *Re-Thinking Housing with Services in Minnesota: Interim Evaluation Report on Demonstration Projects on Affordable Housing with Services for Older Persons*. St. Paul, MN: Department of Human Services.

Kane, R. A., Kane, R.L., & Ladd, R.C. (1998). *The Heart of Long-Term Care*. New York: Oxford University Press.

Morris, J., Gutkin, C., Ruchlin, H., & Sherwood, S. (1990). Aging in place: A longitudinal example. In D. Tilson (Ed.), *Aging in Place: Supporting the Frail Elderly in Residential Environments* (pp. 25-52). Glenview, IL: Scott, Foresman.

Niesz, H. & Cohen, R. (2002, October 4). *Acts Affecting Seniors* (OLR Research Report No. 2002-R-0800). Hartford, CT: State of Connecticut Office of Legislative Research, Connecticut General Assembly.

Niesz, H. (2002, October 11). *2002 Private Assisted Living Pilot Legislation* (OLR Research Report No. 2002-R-0854). Hartford, CT: State of Connecticut Office of Legislative Research, Connecticut General Assembly. Retrieved November 12, 2003, from: *http://www.cga.state.ct.us/2002/olrdata/rpt/2002-R-0854htm*

P.A. 00-2, June Special Session. *An Act Concerning Programs and Modifications Necessary to Implement the Budget Relative to the Department of Social Services*. Retrieved November 12, 2003, from: http://www.cga.state.ct.us/2000/act/pa/2000PA-00002-R00HB-06002SS2-PA.htm

Rabins, P., Black, B., German, P., Roca, R., McGuire, M., Brant, L., & Cook, J. (1996). The prevalence of psychiatric disorder in elderly residents in public senior housing. *Journal of Gerontology*, *51A* (6), M319-M324.

Redfoot, D.L., & Pandya, S.M. (2002). *Before the Boom: Trends in Long-Term Supportive Services for Older Americans*. Washington, DC: AARP Public Policy Institute.

Ryan, M.S. (2002a, March). *Developing a true continuum of long-term care*. Symposium conducted at the Connecticut Assisted Living Association Conference. Hartford, CT.

Ryan, M.S. (2002b, March). *Long-term care alternatives*. Symposium conducted at the Connecticut Assisted Living Association Conference, Hartford, CT.

Schalock, R.L., DeVries, D, & Lebsack, J. (1999). Enhancing Quality of Life. In S. Herr & G. Weber (Eds.), *Aging, Rights, and Quality of Life: Prospects for Older*

People with Developmental Disabilities (pp. 81-92). Baltimore: Paul H. Brookes Publishing Company.

Schlesinger, L., & Morris, J. (1982). Characteristics of public housing clients. In J. Morris, S. Sherwood & L. Schlesinger (Eds.), *Serving the Vulnerable Elderly in Massachusetts: The Role of the Commonwealth's Home Care Corporation* (pp. 101-108). Report submitted to the Massachusetts Department of Elder Affairs.

Schuetz, J. (2003, January). *Affordable Assisted Living: Surveying the Possibilities.* Harvard University: Joint Center of Housing Studies.

Sheehan, N.W. (1992). *Successful Administration of Senior Housing: Working with Elderly Residents.* Newbury Park, CA: Sage Publications.

Sheehan, N.W. (1993, March). *The Resident Services Coordinator Model in Federally Assisted Senior Housing: A Final Report.* Storrs: University of Connecticut.

Sheehan, N.W. (1999, October). *Assisted Living Services in Congregate Housing: A Final Report from the Assisted Living Services Pilot Program at St. Jude Common.* Storrs: University of Connecticut.

Sheehan, N.W., & Mahoney, K. (1984). *Connecticut's Elderly Living in Public Senior Housing.* Report submitted to the Gerontological Society of America, Washington, DC.

Sheehan, N.W. & Oakes, C.E. (2003a). Bringing Assisted Living Services into Congregate Housing: Residents' Perspectives. *The Gerontologist, 43,* 766-770.

Sheehan, N.W. & Oakes, C.E. (2003b, November). *Combining Housing and Services: Bringing Assisted Living into State-Funded Congregate Housing.* Paper presented at the Annual Meeting of the Gerontological Society of America, San Diego, CA.

Spector, W.D., Shaffer, T. J., Hodlewsky, R. T. et al. (2000, June 20-21). *Future Directions for Community-Based Long-Term Care Health Services Research: Expert Meeting Summary* (AHRQ Publication No. 02-0022). Rockville, MD: Agency for Healthcare Research and Quality.

State of Connecticut. (2003, December 3). *Balancing the System: Working Towards Real Choice for Long-Term Care in Connecticut.* (Final Report to the General Assembly).

State of Connecticut (2002, March). *Choices Are for Everyone: Continuing the Movement Toward Community-Based Supports in Connecticut.* Hartford, CT: Department of Social Services.

State of Connecticut (1999, January). *Long-Term Care Plan. A Report to the General Assembly.* Hartford, CT: Long-Term Care Planning Committee.

State of Connecticut. (2001, January). *Long-Term Care Plan: A Report to the General Assembly.* Hartford, CT: Connecticut Long-Term Care Planning Committee.

State of Connecticut (October 11, 2002). 2002 *Private Assisted Living Legislation* (2202-R-0854). Hartford, CT: Office of Legislative Research.

Tilson, D. & Fahey, C. (1990). Introduction. In D. Tilson (Ed.), *Aging in Place: Supporting the Frail Elderly in Residential Environments* (pp. xv-xxxiii). Glenview, IL: Scott, Foresman.

U.S. Census Bureau (2000). Results of the U.S. Census. Washington, D. C.: Author.

U.S. General Accounting Office Report to Congressional Requester (1999, April). *Assisted Living: Quality of Care and Consumer Protection Issues in Four States* (GAO/HEHS-99-27). Washington, DC: U.S. General Accounting Office.

U.S. Department of Housing and Urban Development (2002, November). *HUD Awards $54.3 Million to Convert Existing Multifamily Housing into Assisted Living Facilities*. Retrieved November 12, 2003, from: *http://www.hud.gov:80/news/ release.cfm?content=pr02-136.cfm*

Wilden, R. & Redfoot, D.L. (2002, January). *Adding Assisted Living Services to Subsidized Housing: Serving Frail Older Persons with Low Incomes*. Washington, DC: AARP Public Policy Institute.

APPENDIX A
Glossary of State Agencies and Programs

State Agencies:	
CHFA	Connecticut Housing Finance Authority
DCF	Department of Children and Families
DECD	Department of Economic and Community Development
DMHAS	Department of Mental Health and Addiction Services
DMR	Department of Mental Retardation
DOT	Department of Transportation
DPH	Department of Public Health
DSS	Department of Social Services
OPM	Office of Policy and Management
OHCA	Office of Health Care Access
P & A	Office of Protection and Advocacy for Persons with Disabilities
Other Agencies and Programs:	
AAA	Area Agency on Aging
ALS	Assisted Living Services
ALSA	Assisted Living Service Agency
CH	Congregate Housing
CHCPE	Connecticut Home Care Program for Elders
CIL	Center for Independent Living
CSH	Corporation for Supportive Housing
CHSP	Congregate Housing Services Program
RHS	Rural Housing Services
SC	Service Coordinator

APPENDIX B
Membership of the LTC Planning Committee and the LTC Advisory Council

LTC Planning Committee	LTC Advisory Council
• Department of Children and Families • Department of Economic and Community Development • Department of Mental Health and Addiction Services • Department of Mental Retardation • Department of Protection and Advocacy for Persons with Disabilities • Department of Public Health • Department of Social Services • Department of Transportation • Human Services Committee • Office of Health Care Access • Office of Policy and Management • Public Health Committee • Select Committee on Aging	• AARP • Alzheimer's Association of Northern Connecticut • American College of Health Care Administrators • Coalition of Presidents of Resident Councils • Commission on Aging • Connecticut Assisted Living Association • Connecticut Association of Area Agencies on Aging • Connecticut Association of Health Care Facilities, Inc. • Connecticut Association of Home Care • Connecticut Association of Not-For-Profit Providers for the Aging • Connecticut Association of Residential Care Homes • Connecticut Community Care, Inc. • Connecticut Council for Persons with Disabilities • Connecticut Hospital Association • District 1199 AFL-CIO • Greater Hartford Legal Assistance Long-Term Care Ombudsmen Program • Long-Term Care Planning Committee • The Family Support Council • Select Committee on Aging ------------------------------ • Non-union home health aide (1) • Person who cares for a person with a disability in a home setting (1) • Personal care attendant (1) • People with disabilities (3)

APPENDIX C
Assisted Living Services Days of Billing by Service Level (October 2003)

	Level 1: 1 - 3 hrs/wk $16.32/day	Level 2: 4 - 8 hrs/wk $31.88/day	Level 3: 9 - 15 hrs/wk $47.53/day	Level 4: 15 +/hrs/wk $66.30/day	Total days
Congregate-ALS	848	711	155	31	1,745
HUD-ALS	315	1,008	258	31	1,616
Private Assisted Living Pilot	116	157	177	220	670

Supportive Housing Initiatives in Arkansas

Debra Tillery

SUMMARY. Arkansas has a significant need for improving the availability of affordable housing with access to supportive services for its large population of elderly and persons with disabilities. Factors that contribute to this need are the high level of poverty, general poor health, low employment rate for persons with disabilities, and the geographic and social isolation problems typical of a rural state. *[Article copies available for a fee from The Haworth Document Delivery Service: 1-800-HAWORTH. E-mail address: <docdelivery@haworthpress.com> Website: <http://www.HaworthPress.com> © 2004 by The Haworth Press, Inc. All rights reserved.]*

KEYWORDS. Long-term care, housing, aging, affordable, public policy, Arkansas, rural, assisted living

Objectives

The purpose of this paper is to examine four separate supportive housing initiatives that have the common goal of creating more housing options for low-income seniors and people with disabilities and the shared themes of co-

---

Debra Tillery, MA, is affiliated with Information Brokering for Long-Term Care, a project of the Center for Home Care Policy & Research of the Visiting Nurse Service of New York.
Funded by the Robert Wood Johnson Foundation.

[Haworth co-indexing entry note]: "Supportive Housing Initiatives in Arkansas." Tillery, Debra. Co-published simultaneously in *Journal of Housing for the Elderly* (The Haworth Press, Inc.) Vol. 18, No. 3/4, 2004, pp. 115-136; and: *Linking Housing and Services for Older Adults: Obstacles, Options, and Opportunities* (eds: Jon Pynoos, Penny Hollander Feldman, and Joann Ahrens) The Haworth Press, Inc., 2004, pp. 115-136. Single or multiple copies of this article are available for a fee from The Haworth Document Delivery Service [1-800- HAWORTH, 9:00 a.m. - 5:00 p.m. (EST). E-mail address: docdelivery@haworthpress.com].

operation, collaboration and innovative combination or "layering" of state and federal funding. The four initiatives are:

1. The *Coming Home* Program, a project funded by the Robert Wood Johnson Foundation to establish affordable assisted living options.
2. *The ARC of Arkansas (Affordable, Accessible Housing for Arkansans with and Without Disabilities)*, a housing initiative that couples low-income tax credits and other conventional funding mechanisms with Historic Preservation Tax Credits to renovate abandoned buildings on the National Register of Historic Places into one-of-a-kind, ADA-accessible affordable housing.
3. *The Area Agencies on Aging (AAAs)* sponsor Affordable Housing with Supportive Services projects whereby AAAs broker and participate in public and private partnerships to build safe, affordable housing for Arkansas residents.
4. *The Arkansas Governor's Supported Housing Task Force*, a collaboration designed to share information and resources in order to develop and implement a comprehensive, effective working Olmstead plan.

Findings

Housing Resources and Funding Mechanisms

- *The state/county entities involved with housing mirror those of many other states.* They include entities in charge of financing, economic development, human services, rehabilitation, local public housing and rural housing.
- *Similarly, the funding mechanisms are a patchwork of federal and state programs* that provide tax credits, loans and loan guarantees, tax-exempt bonds and rental assistance to stimulate the development and occupancy of low-income housing units.

The Coming Home Program

- Implementation of the Coming Home Program was greatly facilitated by technical assistance and short-term predevelopment financing provided by the NCB Development Corporation as part of the RWJF initiative. This assistance helped with real estate issues and financing plans, with coordination of Medicaid payments for health, social and personal care services, and with identification of federal, state and private financing mechanisms. The short-term financing was used to cover initial development costs before other funding sources became available.
- An important outcome of the Coming Home Program was the passage of state legislation that recognizes assisted living as a new category of li-

censed long-term care facility requiring a Permit of Approval (POA) or certificate of need.

- The processes involved in passing the assisted living facility (ALF) legislation and in promulgating the necessary regulations were highly political, involving legislators, lobbyists for the nursing home and residential care facility associations, and advocacy groups representing the interests of elders and people with disabilities. The result was that minimal modifications in physical plant or amenities are required to convert to ALF status, that residential care facilities (RCFs) are permitted to continue to use the term "assisted living" to promote their services, and that two levels of ALF were established–one that differs only slightly from current RCFs and one that can accept people with more complex medical needs.
- So far one ALF has been opened as a result of the Coming Home Program, while two more are underway.

The ARC of Arkansas

- The ARC attributes the success of their projects to working with an experienced development company, the First Security Vanadis Capital, LLC, a pioneer in community development finance and in reintroducing multi-family living to the urban core of once-populated downtown neighborhoods.
- The natural mix of residents has resulted in about one third of the residents in their buildings being persons with disabilities.
- An added bonus has been the attraction of more personal care attendants to serve residents with disabilities because the area is safe and neighbors see the need and apply for the jobs. The ARC also subsidizes the rent of staff who live at each property and assist the people with disabilities who are clients of the ARC.

Arkansas Area Agencies on Aging

- Supportive housing is considered high-risk and costly due to the complicated application and funding structure, the mandatory up-front expenses (for Section 202, applicants must certify one percent of the total costs of the development), and the non-recoverable expenses (environmental studies, etc.). In addition, administrative tasks associated with managing the units use valuable agency resources and staff time.
- Despite these challenges, the AAA involvement with housing is seen to meet an important need for vulnerable populations, provides the agen-

cies with positive publicity, and creates jobs in the community. Five of the eight Arkansas AAAs now offer low-income housing funded through Housing and Urban Development (HUD) and the Arkansas Development Finance Authority (ADFA) in recognition of the critical need for supportive housing for the elderly.

The Governor's Task Force on Supported Housing

- The work of the Task Force proceeded with the help of the Technical Assistance Collaborative (TAC), a non-profit organization based in Boston whose purpose is to assist states and localities to develop housing strategies. TAC was charged with assessing the federal and state housing resources in Arkansas and helping the Task Force develop viable recommendations.
- The Task Force made nine major recommendations:

1. Designate 10% of the HOME Investment Partnerships Program allocation or one million dollars for bridge tenant-based rental subsidies to be used for people qualifying for Medicaid waiver services (approximately 7,000 participants).
2. Develop Community Development Block Grant (CDBG) funding to support affordable housing.
3. Request the Arkansas Department of Economic Development to reserve 19% or $2.5 million for capital financing for renovation and new construction for the production of supportive housing in the state.
4. Seek partnerships between the Arkansas State Department of Human Services (DHS) and the Arkansas Rehabilitation Services in the area of HUD McKinney Act grant funds that are targeted for homeless *Olmstead*-protected individuals moving from institutions to permanent housing.
5. Partner with local Public Housing Authorities to obtain Section 8 vouchers.
6. Dedicate one staff person to oversee implementation of a statewide supportive housing initiative to coordinate housing activity between the DHS, Arkansas Rehabilitation Services and the ADFA.
7. Create a Housing Trust Fund for affordable housing initiatives through allocating a portion of an existing annual fee on building activities.
8. Begin state efforts to coordinate other state and federal agencies under the President's New Freedom Initiative.
9. Propose a pilot program in one urban and one rural community for the purpose of transitioning individuals from institutions into the community.

- Task Force activities have had a systemic impact on the state. Largely based on the high visibility of a gubernatorial selected committee, both public and private awareness of housing issues has been greatly advanced. In addition, definitive actions have been taken to implement a number of the recommendations.

Policy Implications

The four Arkansas supportive housing initiatives follow a common theme of cooperation and education in order to achieve common goals. Each of these initiatives required state agencies, community groups, local organizations and advocates to navigate the complexities of funding resources, housing development, and potential resident needs together. A major success for all of the initiatives was working together to successfully access low-Income Housing Tax Credits from ADFA. While the coordination and combination of tax credits with other funding was challenging and indeed complex, the end result is that the elderly and persons with disabilities will be able to maintain their independence while benefiting from affordable housing with supportive services.

The *Coming Home* initiative encouraged identification of legislative and regulatory barriers to affordable assisted living in Arkansas. It provided DHS an incentive to produce a blueprint for expanding state law to recognize assisted living as a viable new housing option and to create a quality management system for program implementation, and provided funding incentives for private developers. The grant also enabled the state to obtain much-needed federal funding to support assisted living services for Medicaid in the various facilities. *Coming Home* was one of many initiatives that demonstrated Arkansas' commitment to the *Olmstead* Decision and the President's New Freedom Initiative.

The ARC of Arkansas and the Arkansas Area Agencies on Aging found ways to partner with communities and private developers to develop local housing proposals and match needs with support service providers and construction.

The Governor's Task Force on Supported Housing brought various groups to the table for mutual education and promotion of affordable, accessible, assistive living alternatives. Improving access and utilization of public/private partnerships is the only way that Arkansas, and by extension most other states, can serve more people in safer, more affordable housing while providing service supports to allow them to maintain their independence in the least restrictive environment.

By establishing strong partnerships between sister state agencies, community groups, local organizations and advocates, Arkansas is able to proudly highlight a number of successful innovations and share these experiences with others.

INTRODUCTION

Following national trends, Arkansas is seeking to create more viable housing options for the elderly and people with disabilities to live meaningful lives in the community. In doing so, it is responding to several forces: the 1999 Supreme Court *Olmstead* Decision,[1] the President's 2001 *New Freedom Initiative,* and the combined voices of cross-disability advocacy coalitions demanding supportive housing and community-based alternatives to institutional placement.[2]

Arkansas has developed a comprehensive array of community-based services and supports for its citizens, using both traditional and innovative designs.[3] A major focus in Arkansas has been to create affordable housing for the elderly that allows them to maintain their independence and "age in place" by being able to access supportive services such as home-delivered meals and transportation to community health providers. The challenge has been to create accessible, reasonably priced housing by combining available funding resources with appropriate, high-quality support services purchased through public funding (Medicaid or Older Americans Act funding). A dedicated alliance of state agencies and decision-makers has worked together to understand and apply various state and federal policy levers and resources to meet this challenge.

Four Examples of Supportive Housing Initiatives

This case study will highlight four of the many recent initiatives to increase the availability of supportive housing options in Arkansas. Each initiative will be discussed in reference to the current state of affairs in Arkansas, which is briefly described in the next section.

1. *The Coming Home Program:* This initiative, sponsored by the Robert Wood Johnson Foundation (RWJF) and NCB Development Corporation to address the senior housing crisis, demonstrates: (1) the state's legislative efforts to create supportive, affordable housing by legitimizing assisted living as a regulated housing/service category, establishing new regulations for operations, and instituting a new permitting procedure; (2) the cooperation of various state agencies committed to understanding, collaborating and creating common goals toward viable supportive housing; (3) the use of Medicaid funding to underwrite the cost of supports to low-income citizens; and (4) the development of broad public support to provide assisted living for low-income seniors.

2. *The ARC of Arkansas (Affordable, Accessible Housing for Arkansans with and Without Disabilities):* The ARC of Arkansas–a statewide organization providing support, housing, advocacy, education and leader-

ship to people with developmental disabilities and their families–has coupled low-income tax credits and other conventional funding mechanisms with Historic Preservation Tax Credits to renovate abandoned buildings on the National Register of Historic Places into one-of-a-kind, ADA accessible affordable housing. This creates more housing options for all.

3. *The Area Agencies on Aging (AAAs):* The AAAs use their resources and professional staff expertise to broker public and private partnerships in order to build safe, affordable housing funded through Housing and Urban Development (HUD) and the Arkansas Development Finance Authority's (ADFA) HOME program and to attract or provide supportive services to these developments. Resources are combined whenever possible to develop common approaches to funding, architectural services and management, thus saving valuable revenue to support operations rather than development costs.

4. *Arkansas Governor's Supported Housing Task Force:* This task force was created in response to the Governor's May 2000 directive to the State Department of Human Services (DHS) and other affected agencies to develop and implement a comprehensive, effective working Olmstead plan.[4] It brought together advocates, governmental entities, and non-profit organizations to make recommendations regarding housing issues for the elderly and people with disabilities. The Task Force, under the direction of Arkansas Rehabilitation Services, determined that the state was critically underutilizing Community Development Block Grant (CDBG) allocations. Among other things, it recommended that the Arkansas Department of Economic Development reserve 10% of its state CDBG funds for capital financing for renovation and new construction for the production of supportive housing.[5]

BACKGROUND ON ARKANSAS

Demographic Overview

Arkansas is a state with a large and growing elderly population, as well as high poverty rates, medically underserved areas, unemployment and rural isolation. Arkansas currently ranks 9th in the U.S. in its percentage of residents 65 and older, with 14.5% of the state's 2.5 million people being 65 and older.[6] Between 1993 and 2000, the number of Arkansans aged 75-84 increased 37% and the number of Arkansans aged 85 years and older increased by 34%.[7] The United States Census Bureau predicts that Arkansas will rank 5th in the percentage of elderly residents by the year 2025, which means that Arkansas's elderly population will more than double in the next 30 years. The Arkansas Medicare-eligible population is projected to rise to 23.9% in 2025.[8]

Recent studies have shown that Arkansans, and particularly the state's elderly, are in poor health, ranking at or near the bottom of key health parameters when compared to other states.[9] In addition, the state ranked 5th in the percentage of citizens 65 and older with mobility limitations during the last census.[10] Arkansas ties Mississippi with the highest poverty rate in the nation (19%); almost 35% of Arkansas elders are poor or near poor.[11] Economic decline is widespread in the southern and eastern regions of Arkansas despite growth in the northwest region. While there is a 77% employment rate for the non-disabled, persons aged 21 to 64 with disabilities have only a 50% employment rate.[12] According to the USDA, 72% of Arkansas is considered rural, exhibiting high degrees of both geographic and social isolation. More often than not, the elderly living in small rural communities are medically underserved. They seek medical care only when they become seriously ill, leading to higher costs of care once treatment is provided.

Housing Resources and Funding Mechanisms

To a large degree, the state/county entities involved with housing mirror most other states:

- *The Arkansas Development Finance Authority (ADFA)* manages the state low-income Housing Tax Credit Program, the HUD HOME Investment Partnerships Program, and the Mortgage Revenue Bond Program. ADFA has successfully operated as the state's housing finance agency since 1977[13] and is the largest issuer of bonds in the state, allocating over $150 million annually.
- *The Arkansas Department of Economic Development (ADED)* administers the state allocation of HUD CDBG funds and coordinates the Consolidated Planning effort required of entities funded by HUD.
- *The Arkansas Department of Human Services (DHS)* controls the HUD McKinney Act funding for a wide range of homeless assistance, including emergency shelter, transitional and permanent housing, and an array of supportive services.
- Statewide, 155 *Public Housing Authorities* administer 21,000 rental subsidies and manage over 8,000 public housing units.
- *The U.S. Department of Agriculture and Rural Housing Service Program* administers home ownership and home repair programs and the multi-family program for construction of units in rural areas. As of 2003, the program has funded construction of over 10,000 units of affordable housing.

- *The Arkansas Rehabilitation Services* manages a *Supported Housing Office* that provides pre-development technical assistance to individuals or agencies interested in exploring low-income housing, and assists individuals with disabilities to locate accessible housing.

Programs that support *low-income housing* in Arkansas include the *Federal and State Low Income Housing Tax Credit Programs (LIHCP)* and the *Affordable Neighborhood Housing Tax Credit Program.* Funding sources for these programs include the HOME Investment Partnership Program, the Federal Home Loan Bank, Rural Development, tax exempt bonds, 4% LIHCP and HUD.

The Arkansas Tax Reform Act of l986 created *Housing Credit* to encourage private sector investment in the construction and rehabilitation of homes for low to moderate-income persons. This Authority allocates funding for low-income tax credits using the *Qualified Allocation Plan (QAP).* Approximately $3 million annually is dedicated to low-income tax credits in Arkansas, generating approximately $27 million for equity in projects. To date, over 11,000 units are operational throughout the state, with over 48 projects (2,000 units) under construction. Over the past three years, ADFA has targeted the elderly and persons with disabilities by assigning extra points to housing for these special groups. In 2000, approximately 40% of all units funded were specifically for the elderly. Assisted living facilities will be added to the category of construction assigned extra points.

The *Affordable Neighborhood Housing Tax Credit* is a state tax credit authorized by ADFA to business firms that provide affordable housing assistance activities to non-profit neighborhood organizations. The amount of the one-time tax credit cannot exceed 30% of the value of the contribution. Allocations are approved through the submission of a detailed project application to ADFA. Assisted living facilities will be eligible for this tax credit. [14]

Federal HOME program funds targeted to low-income residents are available through HUD's *Rental Housing Programs, Homeowner Housing Programs* and *Tenant Based Rental Assistance Program.* Since l992, the HOME Program has provided over $6.2 million to assist in the construction of approximately 250 HOME-assisted rental housing units for the elderly with an average cost per unit of $25,000. Funding is disbursed using a competitive application process and evaluated by the ADFA and the Housing Review Committee Board on capacity, housing need, ability to leverage other funds, and readiness. During the next state fiscal year, Arkansas will receive over $11 million under this program. Over 70% of these funds will be specifically dedicated to the development of new or the renovation of existing rental and purchased housing.

AFFORDABLE ASSISTED LIVING:
THE COMING HOME PROGRAM

Assisted living, residential care and continuing-care communities are expensive LTC options beyond the reach of most seniors. The primary focus of the Robert Wood Johnson Foundation (RWJF) *Coming Home* Program is to create affordable assisted living, especially for people with limited means living in rural areas. This program is designed to help states develop affordable assisted living by:

- Creating a supportive policy environment
- Demonstrating the viability of financing ALFs
- Building partnerships among state agencies, housing developers and nonprofit providers

In January 2001, Arkansas received one of nine *Coming Home* grants to create an assisted living model to serve low-income seniors (including those on Medicaid with income at or less than 300% of SSI or $545 per month) by reducing shelter payments to about $350-$400 per month and funding necessary supportive services through Medicaid. The initiative involved combining a comprehensive service package under a Medicaid §1915(c) Home- and Community-Based Services (HCBS) Waiver with other available funding sources specific to housing or with revolving loans. Funding was provided by RWJF to support state staff to develop, implement and manage the program, and technical assistance was provided by NCB Development Corporation (NCBDC), a national non-profit organization whose mission is to improve the lives of low-income individuals, families and communities. *The desired end result was the provision of safe, affordable housing with health, social, and personal care services for persons with limited income and resources.*

The NCBDC approach included: providing assistance with real estate issues and financing plans; working with state agencies to coordinate Medicaid payments for health, social and personal care services; and identifying federal, state and private financing mechanisms. In addition, NCBDC provided short-term predevelopment financing to cover initial development costs. Developers of assisted living facilities were also encouraged to access low-interest public financing to significantly lower the rent needed to service a conventional mortgage.

The Arkansas Development Finance Authority (ADFA), through collaboration with the DHS, played a significant role by encouraging flexible use of government funds to leverage community support for new construction in underserved areas of the state. The two state agencies overcame differences in history, language and political direction to reassess their objectives and develop a common approach to affordable, supportive housing. This collaboration resulted in a greater understanding and mutual appreciation of agency objectives and culminated in a dedicated allocation or set-aside specifically to promote construction of assisted living facilities under the *Coming Home* initiative. Through 2003 ADFA has allocated $12 million in tax credits for affordable assisted living in Arkansas. This is equivalent to $4.46 per capita. (A $4.46 per capita allocation in the State of New York would equal over $84 million.)

Assisted Living Recognized as a New Category of LTC Facility

In 2001, Arkansas passed legislation to recognize assisted living as a new category of licensed LTC facility that: provides a level of care intermediate between residential care and skilled nursing care, is regulated under state law; and requires a Permit of Approval (POA) or certificate of need. The stated purposes of Act 1230 of 2001, the Arkansas Assisted Living Act, include promoting *"the availability of appropriate services for elderly persons and adults with disabilities in the least restrictive and most homelike environment"* and encouraging *"the development of innovative and affordable facilities particularly for persons with low to moderate income."*[15] The act defines assisted living and describes both the services that can be provided (assistance with housing, meals, laundry, socialization, transportation, personal services and limited nursing services) and those that cannot (skilled nursing care prescribed by a physician and requiring 24-hour nursing supervision).

In response to considerable pressure from lobbyists for the Arkansas Residential Care Assisted Living Association, the bill also includes provisions to allow residential care facilities (RCFs) to convert to assisted living facilities (ALFs), with minimal physical plant and amenities modifications. In addition, existing facilities licensed as RCFs are permitted to continue to use the term "assisted living" to promote their services. The legislation also requires DHS to apply for a Section 1915(c) waiver *"to increase access to services in assisted living facilities by raising Medicaid income and resource limits to the maximum eligibility level of other home and community-based waivers in effect."* It even includes a specific exemption from the requirement for a POA for one new facility to serve as a pilot project *"in order to take advantage of a Robert Wood Johnson Foundation grant."*

Prior to Act 1230, the state recognized and licensed only RCFs, Intermediate Care Facilities for the Mentally Retarded, nursing facilities, and Adult Day Service Facilities. State laws prohibited RCFs from admitting persons meeting nursing home admission criteria and from offering nursing services to residents. In the absence of public funding to support these facilities, RCF residents pay privately for room and board with their SSI and/or their SSA income. Supportive services are provided to those RCF residents who meet Medicaid income and resource eligibility for State Plan Personal Care services. These services are provided in some cases by the RCF owners, who may be licensed Medicaid Providers of State Plan Personal Care services. Upscale RCFs, promoted to the public as "assisted living facilities," are available only to those with moderate or better incomes.

The process of promulgating regulations governing assisted living facilities and finalizing a methodology to cover granting of POAs for assisted living facilities continued through November of 2003. It involved legislators, representatives of state agencies, lobbyists for the nursing home and RCF associations, and advocacy organizations representing the interests of the elderly and people with disabilities. In response to intense pressure from industry lobbyists, two levels of assisted living facilities were created by regulation. The Level 1 ALF is based on a social model and differs only slightly from RCFs. Facilities currently permitted as RCFs were encouraged to convert to Level 1 ALFs. Level 2 ALFs, which offer medication administration and nursing care, can accept persons with more complex medical needs who meet the criteria for nursing facility admission.

Service Package Created Through a Waiver Program

The state submitted a Section 1915(c) waiver application to the Centers for Medicare and Medicaid Services (CMS) to obtain funding for the service package under Medicaid. The waiver, which was approved in mid-2002 to serve no more than 200 individuals at one time,[16] allows Medicaid eligibles over age 21 who meet nursing home admission criteria to receive services reimbursed by Medicaid in licensed Level II ALFs. The waiver also allowed individuals having an income at or less than 300% of SSI to be included as part of the eligible population.

Under the waiver, the facility must provide or contract for 24-hour staff supervision; three meals per day, 7 days per week, with the availability of special diets; other support services (include assistance with both activities and instrumental activities of daily living); and limited nursing care. As of the winter of 2003, daily rates for Medicaid assisted living reimbursement ranged from $38.40 per day per resident to $48.56 per day per resident.[17] Each individual on the waiver may use State Plan Medicaid services (i.e., home health services, durable medical equipment, therapy services, etc.) to the degree that the service does not duplicate those offered under the assisted living package. The waiver also allows each eligible individual to receive three prescription drugs beyond the Medicaid State Plan Prescription Drug Program's monthly benefit limit and to exercise the option to consult with a pharmacist. These options are in addition to the daily per diem rate.

The Medicaid eligible is allowed to retain $50.00 per month for personal expenses. The remainder of his or her income is divided between room and board expenses (generally the SSI amount) and applied to the cost of the waiver service. For example, a waiver eligible person receives assisted living services totaling $1,764.30 per month and receives a $900 Social Security check each month. After $50 is deducted for personal needs and $502 is deducted for rent, the $348 that remains from the Social Security check is applied to the cost of the waiver services. Medicaid reimburses the remaining amount of the cost of the waiver services ($1,416.30).

An Affordable Assisted Living Facility Is Established

In December 2002, one of the nation's first truly affordable assisted living facilities, the Gardens at Osage Terrace, opened in Bentonville, Arkansas.[18] This facility, which was exempted from the requirement for a POA under Act 1230 of 2001, exclusively serves Medicaid eligibles and individuals at or below 60% of the area median income. The facility was funded with assistance from multiple government agencies and represents collaboration between NCBDC of Bentonville/Bella Vista, the ADFA, and the DHS Division of Aging and Adult Services. The ADFA provided $300,000 in HUD HOME Investment Partnership funds, and awarded Low-Income Housing Tax Credits totaling over $2.2 million. Other partners included the Federal Home Loan Bank of Dallas ($450,000 grant), Community Care Foundation ($187,000 grant), and the Arvest Bank of Bentonville ($750,000).[19]

In May of 2003, two additional projects, which will be built in extremely poor communities, were awarded federal low-income housing tax credits under the *Coming Home* initiative—Fruit of the Spirit in College Station near Little Rock and Whispering Knoll in Pine Bluff. Both projects will serve predominantly low-income, Medicaid-eligible elderly—a population that has substantially lower income than the minimum income required for a tax credit project. Approximately $5 million in federal low income housing tax credits in total were allocated to developers of affordable housing in Arkansas. Ten percent of the allocation went to these two *Coming Home* projects.[20] Unlike the Bentonville facility that was exempt from the requirement for a POA, both of these facilities applied for and received POAs under the new Health Services Permitting Commission's Assisted Living Methodology. This regulation gives priority for new construction to applicants who demonstrate that "their application will serve low-income elderly residents" and can "provide documentation of pending application with Arkansas Finance Authority for tax credit." Both will create 40 assisted living units and partner with local senior care providers to meet the service needs of the residents.

The Arkansas *Coming Home* collaboration formally ended in January 2004. Its success should not be judged by numbers alone–either number of facilities or number of Medicaid eligibles served (about 50 at the Bentonville facility)–but by the fact that this initiative helped change the face of LTC in Arkansas *by proving that it is possible to overcome barriers to affordable assisted living through innovative strategies of "layering" various financing mechanisms with tax credits.*

THE ARC OF ARKANSAS

The unique housing initiatives of the ARC of Arkansas are an essential part of their overarching goal of integrating persons with disabilities into the community. They provide quality affordable, accessible housing for Arkansans with and without disabilities. The ARC's housing projects are all renovated historic buildings donated to the organization and located along regular bus lines that feature Universal Design standards to attract and accommodate all persons.

Creating Housing from Historic Buildings

For their first project in 1998, the ARC used Low Income Tax Credits, funds from the ADFA HOME program and the Federal Home Loan Bank, Historic Preservation Tax Credits, and a Landmark Grant from the Historic Preservation Trust to create Trinity Court Place Apartments, a one-of-a-kind, 22-unit independent living facility for low- to moderate-income disabled residents and their families.[21] Their next two projects, also fully compliant with Americans with Disabilities Act (ADA) requirements, similarly relied on Low Income and Historic Preservation Tax Credits. Eastside Lofts, a renovation of the Eastside High School building that was built in 1903 and is on the National Register of Historic Places, opened in January 2002. The Eastside Lofts development converted the main building into 41 affordable housing units, advertised in the January 2004 issue of Apartment Finder as one-to three-bedroom units renting for $220-$925 per month to individuals whose annual income meets affordable housing qualifications. Westside Lofts, a similar 43-unit renovation of the Westside Junior High School built in 1917, opened in December 2003. Following a demographic study to determine need, their latest project targets persons 55 and older in a community with a need for retirement housing. The ARC currently has four properties with 131 rental units. The natural mix of residents has resulted in about one third of the residents in their buildings being persons with disabilities.

The ARC attributes the success of their projects to working with an experienced development company, the First Security Vanadis Capital, LLC, a pioneer in community development finance and in reintroducing multi-family living to the urban core of once-populated downtown neighborhoods. In addition, ARC staff educate the developers and management company on universal design and the specific needs of the elderly and persons with disabilities, and are sensitive to the wishes of their communities. Historic preservation advocates applaud saving these unique structures, neighborhood groups see the projects as stabilizing forces that revitalize the community and provide wonderful housing and services, and people with disabilities are welcomed in the community. An added bonus has been the attraction of more personal care attendants to serve residents with disabilities because the area is safe and neighbors see the need and apply for the jobs. The ARC also subsidizes the rent of staff who live at each property and assist the people with disabilities who are clients of the ARC.

AFFORDABLE HOUSING WITH SUPPORTIVE SERVICES: THE AREA AGENCIES ON AGING

For a number of years, five of the eight Arkansas Area Agencies on Aging (AAAs) have offered low-income housing funded through HUD and ADFA in recognition of the critical need for supportive housing for the elderly. Supportive housing is considered high-risk and costly due to the complicated application and funding structure, the mandatory up-front expenses (for Section 202, applicants must certify one percent of the total costs of the development), and the non-recoverable expenses (environmental studies, etc.). In addition, administrative tasks associated with managing the units use valuable agency resources and staff time. However, despite these challenges, the AAA involvement with housing is seen to meet an important need for vulnerable populations, provide the agencies with positive publicity, and create jobs in the community.

Developing Affordable Elderly Housing in Rural Arkansas

The AAA of Southwest Arkansas has made significant progress in developing affordable, accessible housing in one of the most rural and economically stressed parts of the state. The agency first became familiar with the funding process for low-income housing when it took over Section 8 housing from a local provider and realized that the original tenant plan only served 20% of the elderly in the area. The agency used case managers to demonstrate the unmet need for elderly housing by identifying potential residents and adding their names to housing waiting lists, and approached the local housing board to modify the tenant plan to include a higher number of elderly and persons with disabilities. Then it utilized funding from ADFA's HOME program, tax credits, and loans from the HUD Home and Private Bank Financing to develop a $1.4 million project for low-income elderly and persons with disabilities aged 62 and older. The funding included $800,000 in tax credits from ADFA and two bank loans for 30 years totaling $300,000 each. To coordinate the availability of funds, the AAA created a bridge account to provide immediate funding to construct the units while awaiting the distribution of ADFA and HUD monies. This innovative housing initiative in an economically depressed area of the state highlighted the need for the AAAs to take an active role in promoting affordable housing options for the elderly.[22]

The White River Area Agency on Aging, located in the north central part of the state, owns and manages 12 HUD Section 202 projects with 188 units and employs about 30 community workers. The occupancy rate is a stable 85%, which suggests that these projects are meeting much of the community need for low-income housing for seniors. The agency provides one on-site maintenance and management staff position that is funded either directly by the AAA or, if available, through the Title V Older Americans Act or the state Older Worker Program. Residents requiring support services receive these from any willing provider in the area, including the AAA. While these projects are viewed as community successes, the AAA has made the decision to target housing with a greater capacity for coordinating services such as assisted living, and is currently exploring funding options to support an assisted living initiative.[23]

The AAA of Southeast Arkansas owns and manages 14 projects with 204 units in its 10 county service area, plus a project outside their region in a county that needed housing but had no other non-profits interested in meeting that need. Although initially the agency did not consider housing as a viable activity, it responded to a profound need for low-income housing in this economically depressed area. No one was making plans to improve the situation until a bank in the area expressed an interest in partnering for a HUD sponsored 501 C III project.

The AAA now works exclusively with HUD Section 202 projects. They use a consultant and an architect who work on contingency to deal with the actual application and design process. The AAA finds the land, goes before the city council or county Quorum Court, deals with variances and codes, and then owns and manages the housing units. Their housing development model always includes a community room and an agency service coordinator on site. One facility also includes an on-site senior center. The clients are eligible for the same services available to persons not living in Section 202 housing. These include transportation, chore, telephone reassurance, home delivered meals and others. The AAA projects developed after 1991 are under the Section 202 program. Those developed prior to 1991 were under the HUD 501 C III program. Under Section 202 the sponsor has "allowables," one of which is land. Criteria for selection include community support, source and type of available in-kind match, how the funds will be spent, etc. For instance, land donated by a county would be a plus for the application because more funds could be spent on developing the structures. Project clients must be age 62 or older and meet income requirements based on the county poverty level and figured at 30% of Adjusted Gross Income after deductions. The resident must be able to do certain tasks such as get out of the facility in case of emergency.[24]

A COLLABORATION DESIGNED TO SHARE INFORMATION AND RESOURCES: GOVERNOR'S TASK FORCE ON SUPPORTED HOUSING

The 1999 Supreme Court *Olmstead* Decision has had profound implications for state planning activities that promote the development of integrated community living for the elderly and people with disabilities. Safe, affordable housing is critical to the development of a comprehensive, effectively working plan for placing people with disabilities in less restrictive settings. For this reason, in the summer of 2001, Governor Mike Huckabee directed the Arkansas Rehabilitation Services to convene stakeholders to identify the barriers and issues surrounding the availability of supportive housing and to develop a planning strategy to eliminate those barriers. Task force members included individuals with expertise in real estate development (both state and federal), DHS administrative staff, service providers, and consumers and family members. The task force divided itself into five working committees to answer key questions about supportive housing:[25]

- *Data*–How many persons will require supportive housing, where do they live currently, and what type of supportive housing units will they want?
- *Housing Partnerships*–How can housing developers, service providers, and consumers work together to develop more supportive housing units?
- *Legislative and Public Awareness*–How can the legislature and the general public learn more about supportive housing needs and resources and the *Olmstead* Decision in Arkansas?

- *Home-Based Modifications*–How can we help those who want to move in with family or remain in their own homes to access financial help to modify their homes with ramps, wider doorways, and bathroom modifications?
- *Assisted Living*–For low-income elderly who do not need nursing home care but do need help with meal preparation and/or medication management, how can we assist in the development of assisted living facilities such as those demonstrated in the *"Coming Home"* program?

The Task Force, which was funded by Arkansas Rehabilitation Services, consulted with the Technical Assistance Collaborative, a non-profit organization based in Boston whose purpose is to assist states and localities to develop housing strategies. This organization had developed an *Olmstead* Housing Plan for the state of Maryland and the District of Columbia.[26] This non-profit firm was charged with assessing the federal and state housing resources in Arkansas and assisting the Task Force to make viable recommendations to the Governor to improve the availability of affordable housing.

Recommendations Made to Promote "Normal Housing" in the Community

The Task Force agreed upon three basic assumptions regarding housing in Arkansas: (1) income is the issue for those seeking housing, not their disability; (2) the elderly and younger persons with disabilities, who are often linked categorically as one group, vary substantially in their housing arrangement preferences; and (3) citizens desire "normal housing" in the community rather than segregated, congregate developments.

The Task Force completed an assessment of the housing needs for Arkansas and developed a number of recommendations for the Governor based on a 3-year time frame (see Table 1).

During the past year definitive action has been taken to promote the tenant-based bridge recommendation. In January 2003, a Request for Proposal (RFP) was released inviting interested parties to participate in an initiative that would utilize HOME funds as an immediate support project for the low-income Medicaid population. The Section 8 Voucher Program would eventually sustain this program. Unfortunately, the RFP failed to attract interested applicants. Arkansas Rehabilitation Services is currently in the process of educating the eight AAAs about this potential opportunity, particularly in rural areas of the state. It is anticipated that a second RFP will be issued in the upcoming months.[28]

TABLE 1. Governor's Task Force Recommendations[27]

1)	Designate 10% of the HOME Investment Partnerships Program allocation or one million dollars for bridge tenant-based rental subsidies to be used for people qualifying for Medicaid waiver services (approximately 7,000 participants). Under this recommendation, HOME funds would be provided immediately, with Section 8 vouchers applied upon completion and approval of the application process.
2)	Develop CDBG funding to support affordable housing. The Task Force determined that Arkansas was critically underutilizing CDBG funding in this area, compared to most states.
3)	Request the Arkansas Department of Economic Development to reserve 19% or $2.5 million for capital financing for renovation and new construction for the production of supportive housing in the state. These funds would be used to leverage HOME Program funds, Low-Income Housing Tax Credits, and USDA funds to increase the production of cross-disability, mixed-income developments.
4)	Seek partnerships between the Arkansas DHS and the Arkansas Rehabilitation Services in the area of HUD McKinney Act grant funds that are targeted for homeless *Olmstead*-protected individuals moving from institutions to permanent housing.
5)	Partner with local Public Housing Authorities to obtain Section 8 vouchers.
6)	Dedicate one staff person to oversee implementation of a statewide supportive housing initiative to coordinate housing activity between the DHS, Arkansas Rehabilitation Services and the ADFA.
7)	Create a Housing Trust Fund for affordable housing initiatives through allocating a portion of an existing annual fee on building activities. This funding would combine with HOME, CDBG, and the Tax Credit Program to generate $2 million in new housing funds. The Trust Fund would be available to low-income individuals with disabilities.
8)	Begin state efforts to coordinate other state and federal agencies under the President's New Freedom Initiative. Of particular interest is the HUD response to the President's call to federal agencies for responsiveness to community living.
9)	Propose a pilot program in one urban and one rural community for the purpose of transitioning individuals from institutions into the community. DHS would direct the pilot effort, which would include active participation by the Public Housing Authorities and would support service providers interested in providing community-based support services.

The Task Force continues to actively monitor the activity of each of the five on-going committees and refine the recommendations for implementation. In addition to the recommendations listed above, each committee has selected specific local activities to promote affordable housing. Examples include:

- Incorporating a formal legislative orientation and continuing education program on supportive housing and disability issues;
- Promoting Alternative Financing Program and ADFA's Homeowner Rehabilitation and Rental Rehabilitation funds for home modifications for persons with disabilities;

- Identifying the issues that motivate private developers to participant in affordable, accessible housing projects; and,
- Ensuring that existing housing development units offer fair and equal treatment to persons with disabilities.

Increased Awareness

Task Force activities have had a systemic impact on the state. Largely based on the high visibility of a gubernatorial selected committee, both public and private awareness of housing issues has been greatly advanced. The Task Force on Supported Housing has brought together individuals–both experts in their fields and consumer and family members–to educate each other on needs, resources and barriers. Committee members closely monitor the activity or lack of activity of state and federal housing agencies to ensure communication and collaboration. While empirical evidence of success has yet to be forthcoming, the Task Force continues to have the active support of the Governor and members committed to improving housing options for Arkansans with disabilities.

LESSONS LEARNED

The four Arkansas supportive housing initiatives follow a common theme of cooperation and education in order to achieve common goals. Each of these initiatives required state agencies, community groups, local organizations and advocates to navigate the complexities of funding resources, housing development, and potential resident needs together. A major success for all of the initiatives was working together to successfully access low-Income Housing Tax Credits from ADFA. While the coordination and combination of tax credits with other funding was challenging and indeed complex, the end result is that the elderly and persons with disabilities will be able to maintain their independence while benefiting from affordable housing with supportive services.

The *Coming Home* initiative encouraged identification of legislative and regulatory barriers to affordable assisted living in Arkansas. It gave DHS an incentive to produce a blueprint for expanding state law to recognize assisted living as a viable new housing option and to create a quality management system for program implementation, and provided funding incentives for private developers. The grant also enabled the state to obtain much-needed federal funding to support assisted living services for Medicaid in the various facilities. *Coming Home* was one of many initiatives that demonstrated Arkansas's commitment to the *Olmstead* Decision and the President's New Freedom Initiative.

The ARC of Arkansas and the Arkansas Area Agencies on Aging found ways to partner with communities and private developers to develop local housing proposals and match needs with support service providers and construction.

The Governor's Task Force on Supported Housing brought various groups to the table for mutual education and promotion of affordable, accessible, assistive living alternatives. Improving access and utilization of public/private partnerships is the only way that Arkansas, and by extension most other states, can serve more people in safer, more affordable housing while providing service supports to allow them to maintain their independence in the least restrictive environment.

By establishing strong partnerships between sister state agencies, community groups, local organizations and advocates, Arkansas is able to proudly highlight a number of successful innovations and share these experiences with others.

NOTES

1. *Olmstead v. L.C.,* June 22, 1999.
2. The Arkansas Olmstead Coalition, Arkansas People First, and Advocates Needed Today (ANTs).
3. Sanderson, Herb, Director, DHS Division of Aging and Adult Services (DAAS). Personal Interview. November 21, 2003.
4. Governor Mike Huckabee to Kurt Knickrehm, Director of DHS, May 17, 2000.
5. Davies, J. (June 2002) "Governor's Task Force on Supported Housing." Report submitted to Governor Mike Huckabee.
6. "The Population in Arkansas" University of Arkansas. Vol.1: No.1, January 2000.
7. University of Arkansas. Vol.1: No.1, January 2000.
8. The Henry J. Kaiser Family Foundation Medicare Chart Book, 2nd ed. (Fall 2001).
9. "Behavior Risk Factor Surveillance System Annual Report." Arkansas Department of Health, February 2002.
10. University of Arkansas. Vol.1: No.1, January 2000.
11. *Arkansas Democrat Gazette,* September 27, 2003.
12. University of Arkansas. Vol.1: No.1, January 2000.
13. ADFA Program. Description and General Information http://accessarkansas.org/adfa/programs/lihtcp.html
14. Crisp, Suzanne. *"Coming Home"* Grant Application. Submitted to the Robert Wood Johnson Foundation October 2000.
15. Act 1230 of 2001. *Arkansas State Legislature.* Arkansas Assisted Living. Spring 2001. http://www.arkleg.state.ar.us/ftproot/acts/2001/htm/act1230.pdf

16. Hecker, Jean. Program Director. Division of Aging and Adult Services. Personal Interview. November 10, 2003.

17. Hecker, Jean. Personal Interview. November 10, 2003.

18. "Arkansas Opens One of the Nation's First True Affordable Assisted Living Residences." Press Release by NCB Development Corporation. 12/10/02 PR Newswire.

19. Jenkens, Robert. "Spotlight on the Coming Home Program." *Housing Fact & Findings.* Vol. 5 No. 3, 2003.

20. "Two Arkansas Coming Home Programs Awarded Low-Income Housing Tax Credits," *Arkansas Democrat Gazette*, May 14, 2003.

21. Personal Interview with Steve Hitt, Executive Director/CEO and Cynthia Stone, Assistant Executive Director, the ARC Arkansas. January 15, 2004.

22. Sneed, David, Executive Director, AAA of Southwest Arkansas. Personal Interview. October 17, 2003.

23. Haas, Ed, Executive Director, White River AAA. Personal Interview. December 8, 2003.

24. Bradshaw, Betty. Executive Director, AAA of Southeast Arkansas. Personal Interview. December 3, 2003.

25. Davies, Jeanette. "Governor's Task Force on Supported Housing Plan." Submitted to Governor Mike Huckabee. June 6, 2002.

26. Davies, Jeanette. June 6, 2002.

27. Davies, Jeanette. June 6, 2002.

28. Davies, Jeanette. June 6, 2002.

Targeting Services to Those Most at Risk: Characteristics of Residents in Federally Subsidized Housing

Donald L. Redfoot

Andrew Kochera

SUMMARY. The budget crises facing many state Medicaid programs have increased interest in the goal of linking services and housing as a way to provide more options to people with disabilities at less cost than institutional care. This article examines some of the premises underlying this interest, especially with respect to linking supportive services and federally subsidized housing for older persons. The first section provides a brief history of the activity in this area. The second section examines the risk factors associated with nursing home admission and how those factors match the characteristics of renters receiving subsidies. The third section focuses specifically on the likelihood that subsidized renters will also become eligible for Medicaid. The fourth section explores the capacity of housing programs to meet the challenges associated with service delivery. Finally, the conclusion examines the implications for public policy decision-makers interested in linking services and housing in order to address the long-term care (LTC) needs of older persons with modest incomes. *[Article copies available for a fee from The Haworth Document Delivery Service: 1-800-HAWORTH. E-mail address: <docdelivery@haworthpress.com> Website: <http://www.HaworthPress.com> © 2004 by The Haworth Press, Inc. All rights reserved.]*

[Haworth co-indexing entry note]: "Targeting Services to Those Most at Risk: Characteristics of Residents in Federally Subsidized Housing." Redfoot, Donald L., and Andrew Kochera. Co-published simultaneously in *Journal of Housing for the Elderly* (The Haworth Press, Inc.) Vol. 18, No. 3/4, 2004, pp. 137-163; and: *Linking Housing and Services for Older Adults: Obstacles, Options, and Opportunities* (eds: Jon Pynoos, Penny Hollander Feldman, and Joann Ahrens) The Haworth Press, Inc., 2004, pp. 137-163. Single or multiple copies of this article are available for a fee from The Haworth Document Delivery Service [1-800-HAWORTH, 9:00 a.m. - 5:00 p.m. (EST). E-mail address: docdelivery@haworthpress.com].

http://www.haworthpress.com/web/JHE
Digital Object Identifier: 10.1300/J081v18n03_06

KEYWORDS. Long-term care, housing, aging, affordable, public policy, Medicaid, low-income, subsidized housing, nursing homes, assisted living

A BRIEF HISTORY

The concept of linking housing and service has been discussed for decades. In 1963, President Kennedy called for the creation of residential facilities "with housekeeping assistance, central food service, and minor nursing from time to time" (U.S. Senate Special Committee on Aging, 1975).

Discussions of linking services with housing, especially in public policy circles, have often emphasized the goal of preventing unnecessary institutionalization. For example, legislation creating the Congregate Housing Services Program (CHSP) in 1978 highlighted the finding that "congregate housing, coordinated with the delivery of supportive services, offers an innovative, proven, and cost-effective means of enabling temporarily disabled or handicapped individuals to maintain their dignity and independence and to avoid costly and unnecessary institutionalization" (Public Law 95-557, 1978). An evaluation of the CHSP in 1987 by the House Select Committee on Aging found that the program was "effective in preventing premature institutionalization" (U.S. House Select Committee on Aging, 1987).

In the years since the enactment of the CHSP, Congress has taken several more steps to promote services in housing with the goal of preventing nursing home placement including:

- reforms to the CHSP with the objective of expanding the program in 1990;
- reforms to the Section 202 Elderly Housing program to enable more service provision (1990);
- authorization of service coordinators in federally subsidized housing (1990, 1992); and,
- authorization of the conversion of some elderly housing projects to provide assisted living services (2000).

In addition, some states have launched programs to target services to the residents of subsidized housing (Wilden and Redfoot, 2002). In some areas, local public housing authorities and sponsors of privately owned subsidized housing have patched together extensive service packages to enable residents to age in place and avoid nursing homes (Wilden and Redfoot, 2002).

CHARACTERISTICS OF SUBSIDIZED RENTERS AND THE RISKS OF NURSING HOME ADMISSION

It is useful to begin by comparing research on the health-related, social, and economic factors that are associated with risk of nursing home admission with research on the characteristics of the 1.8 million residents aged 62 and older in subsidized housing programs.[1] Some of the risk factors are fairly obvious, such as age and disability, while others may be less obvious, such as gender, income, and marital status. These data show that housing subsidy programs serving older persons have very efficiently, if inadvertently, targeted those at heightened risk of nursing home admission. For each of the factors examined below, older tenants in federally subsidized housing are at much higher risk than the rest of the older population.

Age

The risks of disability and nursing home use rise dramatically with advancing age. The likelihood of severe disability increases from 1 in 30 for those aged 65 to 74, to 1 in 10 for those aged 75 to 84, and to 1 in 3 for those aged 85 and older (Stucki and Mulvey, 2000). According to the 1999 National Nursing Home Survey, there were 10.8 nursing home residents per thousand population aged 65 to 74, 43.0 per thousand aged 75 to 84, and 182.5 per thousand aged 85 and older (National Center for Health Statistics, 2002). Among persons aged 95 and older, 43.1 percent are receiving institutional care (Spector et al., 2000).

According to data from the 2002 American Communities Survey,[2] roughly half of older renters receiving subsidies are aged 75 and older, which is a much higher percentage than for homeowners and slightly higher than for renters not receiving subsidies (see Table 1).

The age-related risk of nursing home admission among residents of subsidized housing may be increasing because it is an aging population. In three waves of national surveys of the Section 202 Elderly Housing Program, the average age of

TABLE 1. Age of Residents Aged 62 and Older by Housing Type, 2002

Age	Owners	Renters, No Subsidy	Renters, With Subsidy	Total
62-74	62.6%	55.4%	50.1%	61.1%
75-84	29.9%	31.2%	36.0%	30.3%
85+	7.5%	13.5%	13.9%	8.6%
Median Age	72	73	74	72

Source: 2002 American Community Survey, Analysis by AARP PPI staff.

residents rose from 72.0 years in 1983, to 73.6 years in 1988, and to 75.0 years in 1999. The oldest projects tend to serve the oldest residents. Among projects built before 1974, the average age of residents was 78.1 years, with 38.6 percent of residents older than 80 years old (Heumann, Winter-Nelson, and Anderson, 2001).

Age and age-related disabilities appear to be major factors in seeking subsidized housing. Section 202 housing managers were asked in the 1999 survey to name the primary reason applicants apply to live in their housing. Support with frailties was cited much more frequently as the primary reason for seeking elderly housing among applicants aged 80 years and older (see Table 2).

Disability

The most obvious risk factor contributing to nursing home admission is disability. Researchers measure disability by ability to perform two types of basic tasks. Measures of activities of daily living (ADL) limitations are related to those actions that are necessary to get through the day and include such activities as dressing, bathing, toileting, transferring from bed to chair, walking, and eating. Measures of instrumental activities of daily living (IADL) limitations are related to managing a household and include such activities as paying bills, using a telephone, and shopping. The higher the level of disability, the higher is the risk of being in an institution. According to the 1999 National Long-Term Care Survey, 5.1 percent of people aged 65 and older with only IADL limitations were in institutions compared to 10.2 percent of those with one to three ADL limitations and 47.0 percent of those with four to six ADL limitations (1999 NLTCS, 2003).

Data from the mid-1990s show that older tenants in subsidized housing report much higher levels of disability than other older renters or homeowners. Although different surveys used somewhat different measures of disability, the pattern from each survey was very similar (see Table 3).

TABLE 2. Needs Influencing the Decision to Move to Section 202 Housing by Age of the Applicant

Age of the Applicant	Financial Assistance	Support with Frailties	Increased Social Contacts	Improved Housing Quality	Improved Security
Under 62	64.8%	9.4%	2.7%	20.0%	3.1%
62-69	64.0%	2.7%	9.1%	16.0%	8.3%
70-79	51.7%	7.7%	11.6%	13.8%	15.2%
80+	48.1%	20.3%	4.3%	10.4%	16.9%

Source: Heumann, Winter-Nelson, and Anderson, 2001.

Although higher levels of ADL limitations are most strongly related to nursing home admission, IADL limitations are also strongly related to increased risk of nursing home placement among public housing residents (Black, Rabins, and German, 1999). Consistent with the earlier research from the mid-1990s, the 2002 American Communities Survey found that older renters receiving subsidies were twice as likely as homeowners to experience the activity limitations and conditions measured in the survey (see Table 4).

TABLE 3. Percentage of Persons Aged 65 and Older Reporting Disabilities by Housing Tenure

	Older Homeowners	Older Unsubsidized Renters	Older Subsidized Renters
Some difficulty with an ADL or IADL (1994-1995 SIPP)	18.8	28.1	40.2
Need help with an ADL or IADL (1995 AHS)	16.2	18.8	31.5

Source: Survey of Income and Program Participation, 1994-1995 (U.S. Census Bureau, 1995),[3] and the American Housing Survey (Department of Housing and Urban Development, 1995); Analysis by AARP Public Policy Institute (PPI).

TABLE 4. Percentage of Persons Aged 62 and Older Reporting Long-Lasting Conditions and Activity Limitations by Housing Type

	Owners	Renters, No Subsidy	Renters, With Subsidy	Total
Vision or Hearing Impairment	13.9	18.5	26.5	15.1
Remembering or Concentrating	8.9	13.7	20.0	10.0
Dressing, Bathing, Getting Around Home	7.5	11.3	17.8	8.4
Going Out to Shop or Visit Doctor	15.0	22.4	32.6	16.8
Walking, Climbing Stairs, Reaching, Lifting, Carrying	26.7	35.8	53.4	29.1
Any of the Above Limitations	37.1	48.0	67.2	40.0

Source: 2002 American Communities Survey, Analysis by AARP PPI staff.

Disability levels among residents in subsidized housing appear to be increasing as this population ages. In the 1999 survey of Section 202 housing, managers estimated that 22 percent of their residents were frail, compared to the 13 percent estimated in the 1988 survey.[4] Much more dramatic were the increases in specific disabilities reported by these managers (see Table 5).

Gender and Marital Status

Older women are at a much higher risk of entering a nursing home than older men. According to the 1999 National Nursing Home Survey, 74.3 percent of nursing home residents aged 65 and older were women (NCHS, 2002), which is virtually identical to the percentage of older residents in subsidized housing who are women (73.9 percent) (American Communities Survey, 2002).[5] Older women are more likely to be in nursing homes for at least two reasons:

1. They have a much higher prevalence of disability than older men, especially at the highest levels of disability.
2. The longer life expectancy among women means that they are more likely to outlive their spouses and, therefore, have less support later in life.

Higher levels of disability among older women were found in the 1999 National Long-Term Care Survey (see Table 6).

TABLE 5. Percent of Residents Having Difficulty Performing Various Activities, as Reported by Manager

	1988 (All Projects)	1999 (All Projects)
Getting out of chairs	11.0	30.5
Getting to and from places	11.4	34.0
Performing personal care	4.9	18.5
Taking prescribed medications	NA	18.9
Preparing meals	5.4	18.7
Finding way into apartment	0.8	1.9
Remembering to do things	4.0	11.2
Doing laundry	6.5	21.3
Doing housekeeping	9.4	26.6
Average of all activities	NA	20.2

Source: Heumann, Winter-Nelson, and Anderson, 2001.

The availability of such support is nearly as important as disability in determining whether a person ends up in a nursing home or not. According to the National Academy on Aging, only seven percent of older persons with LTC needs who have family supports are living in nursing homes compared to 50 percent of those who have no family supports (Stone, 2000). Older women are not only more likely to experience a disability; they are also less likely to have informal supports from a spouse when faced with disability. As a result, there is a strong relationship between marital status and residing in an institution (see Table 7).

In addition, older renters in subsidized housing are far less likely to have a spouse present than older homeowners or other older renters (see Table 8).

More research is needed to identify the network of relatives and friends who provide informal support to residents in subsidized housing, though some studies suggest that such support is very weak. An evaluation of participants in the CHSP found that one in three participants had no living children (U.S. House Select Committee on Aging, 1987). A more recent survey of 573 older residents in subsidized housing in Florida also found that one-third of the respondents had no one to turn to for help in the event they were sick or disabled and another 16 percent could rely on someone for help only now and then (Golant, 1999).

TABLE 6. Percentage of Persons 65 and Older with Various Levels of Disability by Gender, 1999

	Men	Women
Any Disability	14.5	23.4
IADLs Only	4.3	5.8
1-3 ADLs	4.5	7.6
4-6 ADLs	5.7	10.0

Source: 1999 National Long-Term Care Survey, Analysis by AARP PPI staff.

TABLE 7. Percentage of Persons Aged 65 and Older Living in Institutions by Marital Status and Level of Disability, 1999

	Married	Widowed	Not Married, Other
Any Disability	11.9	29.8	32.7
IADLs Only	1.7	5.5	12.4
1-3 ADLs	3.9	12.8	15.8
4-6 ADLs	27.2	54.9	62.2

Source: 1999 National Long-Term Care Survey, Analysis by AARP PPI staff.

TABLE 8. Percentage of Persons Aged 62 and Older in Various Living Arrangements by Housing Tenure, 2002

	Married, Spouse Present	Living Alone	Other
Owners	62.2	22.6	15.2
Renters, No Subsidy	33.0	46.4	20.6
Renters, With Subsidy	15.6	73.4	11.0

Source: 2002 American Communities Survey, Analysis by AARP Public Policy Institute.

Race and Ethnicity

Past studies have shown that the use of nursing homes by older Blacks, Hispanics, and Asian Americans has been substantially lower than that of non-Hispanic Whites (Wallace et al., 1998; Damon-Rodriguez et al., 1994; Dilworth-Anderson et al., 2002). This historic pattern has recently changed dramatically for Blacks. Trend data from the National Nursing Home Survey (NNHS) indicate that nursing home utilization rates have declined substantially among older Whites, while they have increased even more substantially among older Blacks. Nursing home utilization is now higher among older Blacks than among older Whites (see Figure 1).

Trend data on Asian Americans and Hispanic Americans are more tenuous because of the small numbers in national surveys. Himes et al. (1996) note that institutional utilization rates are much lower among Hispanics and Asians than among Whites or Blacks. Using 1990 Census data on persons aged 60 and older, they found that the institutionalization rate was 3.3 percent for Whites, 3.1 percent for Blacks, 2.3 percent for Native Americans, 1.6 percent for Hispanics, and 1.2 percent for Asians. They argued that the lower rates for Native Americans, Asians, and Hispanics strongly suggest a cultural preference for family caregiving. Very likely, language barriers and the lack of culturally sensitive services have also contributed to low utilization rates.

A combination of factors has undoubtedly contributed to the counter-trends observed between older Whites and Blacks. Declining discrimination against racial and ethnic minorities may have increased access to nursing home services. Older Blacks are somewhat more likely to have high levels of disabilities–13.7 percent of older Blacks had two or more ADL limitations compared to 11.7 percent of older Whites according to the 1999 National Long-Term Care Survey (NLTCS, 2003). Older Blacks are also much less likely to be living with a spouse than older Whites, and older Black men are more likely than

FIGURE 1. Nursing Home Residents per Thousand Population (Age-Adjusted*) by Race and Selected Years, 1973-74 to 1999

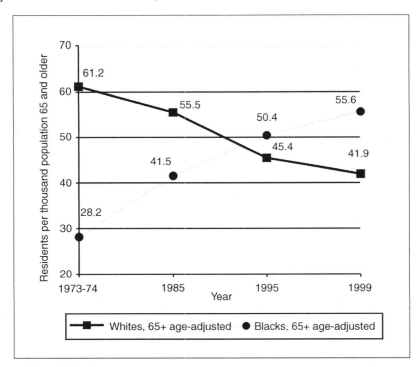

* Note: Age-adjusted by the direct method to the year 2000 population standard using the following three age groups: 65-74, 75-84, and 85 years and older.
Source: The National Nursing Home Survey 1973-74, 1985, 1995, and 1999, National Center for Health Statistics, 2001. Prepared by AARP Public Policy Institute, Redfoot and Pandya, 2002.

their White counterparts to be living alone (see Table 9). These data also show that older Whites are much less likely to live with others (primarily relatives) than other racial/ethnic groups.

Economic status has also played a role in the trends in nursing home utilization among older Whites and Blacks. The number of nursing home residents paying privately declined by 25.2 percent between 1985 and 1999 despite the large increase in the older population (Redfoot and Pandya, 2002). Bishop (1999) argues that this decline can in large part be explained by the growth of supportive housing options like assisted living. Few racial and ethnic minorities have been served by private pay assisted living; a nationally representative study of "high service or high privacy assisted living facilities" found that 98.7 percent of the residents were white (Hawes et al., 2000). The greater reliance on public programs, especially Medicaid, to pay for LTC services may mean that older Blacks have fewer choices other than nursing homes (see Table 10).

In short, older Blacks are at higher risk of nursing home admission than older Whites because they have higher rates of disability, lower rates of living with a spouse, and higher reliance on Medicaid with its bias toward nursing home services. Some of the same social and economic factors have undoubtedly contributed to the higher proportion of older Blacks and other minorities living in subsidized housing. Although older Whites represent more than two-thirds of the older residents in subsidized housing, older Blacks, Hispanics, Asians, and Native Americans all have disproportionately high percentages of subsidized renters. For example, older Blacks represent 8.5 percent of all older households but 21.3 percent of all older renters who receive subsidies (see Table 11).

TABLE 9. Percentage of Persons 65 and Older in Various Living Arrangements by Gender and Race/Ethnicity, 1998

	Men			Women		
	With Spouse	Alone	With Others	With Spouse	Alone	With Others
Whites	74.3	17.0	8.7	42.4	41.3	16.4
Blacks	53.5	24.9	21.6	24.3	40.8	34.9
Asian/ Pac. Isl.	72.0	6.6	21.4	41.3	21.2	37.5
Hispanic	66.8	14.0	19.3	36.9	27.4	35.6
Total	72.6	17.3	10.0	40.7	40.8	18.5

Source: Online data compiled from the March Current Population Survey by the Administration on Aging (2004).

TABLE 10. Primary Source of Payment Among Nursing Home Residents by Race, 1999

	Private	Medicare	Medicaid	Other
White	26.5%	14.7%	56.2%	2.7%
Black	4.9%	15.2%	75.7%	4.3%

Source: 1999 National Nursing Home Survey (NCHS, 2002), Analysis by AARP PPI staff.

Income and Assets

Income is an important risk factor related to LTC services in two ways:

1. Older persons with lower incomes are more likely to experience disabilities; and,
2. Medicaid eligibility is determined by income and assets.

Data from the 1999 National Long-Term Care Survey show the strong relationship between income and disability among people aged 65 and older (see Table 12).

By targeting assistance to renters with low incomes, housing programs are also targeting a population that is at a heightened risk of disability. Eligibility for housing assistance varies somewhat depending upon the funding program

TABLE 11. Percentage of Select Racial and Ethnic Groups Among Persons Aged 62 and Older by Housing Tenure, 2002[6]

	Owners	Renters, No Subsidy	Renters, With Subsidy	Total
White	88.7	79.0	69.2	86.5
Black or African American	7.1	13.0	21.3	8.5
Spanish/Hispanic/Latino	4.9	10.3	11.5	5.9
Asian	2.6	4.5	5.2	2.9
American Indian Alaskan or Hawaiian Native	0.9	1.3	1.7	1.0
Other	1.6	3.8	4.5	2.0

Source: 2002 American Communities Survey, Analysis by AARP PPI staff.

TABLE 12. Percentage of Persons Aged 65 and Older Living in the Community Experiencing Different Levels of Disability by Income Quartile, 1999

	Lowest Quartile	Middle Two Quartiles	Highest Quartile
Any Disability	24.5	14.8	8.8
IADL Only or 1 ADL	12.1	7.6	4.4
2 or More ADLs	12.4	7.2	4.4

Source: 1999 National Long-Term Care Survey based on Urban Institute analysis for AARP PPI

and the location of the housing, but in general housing assistance is limited to those who have incomes below 50 percent of the local median income. In 1997 the median income for older households in public housing was $7,451; for project-based Section 8 it was $8,227; and for other programs it was $10,669 (Department of Housing and Urban Development, 1999). The 2002 American Communities Survey found that the median household income for residents in subsidized housing aged 62 and older was $10,450 compared to $22,700 for unsubsidized renters and $36,700 for older homeowners (American Communities Survey, 2002).

Since assets are often used to pay for services, they are an important factor in determining which options are available in the event of a disability. Medicaid is the primary payer for LTC services for people with low incomes and has strict asset limits, usually $2,000 excluding home equity and other basic necessities. Homeowners have far higher levels of assets than renters, even when home equity is excluded (see Table 13).

MEDICAID RISK AMONG SUBSIDIZED RENTERS

The desire to limit Medicaid expenditures by providing lower cost alternatives to nursing homes has driven much of the discussion about linking housing and services. Declining numbers of residents paying privately in nursing homes and growing numbers using private pay assisted living and other options suggest the possibility that linking housing and services could have similar effects for older people who are unable to pay privately. Whether or not

TABLE 13. Net Worth of Households Aged 62 and Older by Housing Tenure, 2000

Total Net Worth	Owners	Renters, No Subsidy	Renters, With Subsidy	Total
Negative or Zero	1%	27%	38%	7%
Under $10,000	2%	37%	50%	10%
$10,000-$49,999	13%	16%	9%	14%
$50,000-$99,000	20%	7%	2%	17%
$100,000-$149,999	15%	4%	1%	12%
$150,000+	49%	9%	0%	40%
Median Net Worth (Excluding Home Equity)	$36,325	$4,298	$234	$28,269

Source: 2000 Survey of Income and Program Participation.

such measures would result in cost-savings for Medicaid is beyond the scope of this article, but an important related question is the degree to which subsidized renters are likely to be eligible or become eligible for Medicaid. Targeting services to older residents in subsidized housing may be more attractive if significant numbers of those residents are likely to become eligible for Medicaid in the event of a disability. This section estimates the overlap between the populations likely to be served by Medicaid and housing subsidy programs.

Although housing subsidy programs and Medicaid both target people with low incomes, their eligibility criteria are very different. Housing subsidy programs are tied to the local area median income (AMI) on the assumption that housing costs differ widely in different areas of the country. Moreover, housing programs differ in their eligibility levels, depending upon when the long-term subsidy contracts were signed with the housing owners or sponsors. In general, most HUD housing subsidy programs today limit participation to renters whose incomes are below 50 percent of the AMI.[7] In contrast, Medicaid eligibility for people aged 65 and older is generally tied to eligibility for the Supplemental Security Income (SSI) program, which in 2004 was limited to individuals with less than $6,624 in annual income and under $2,000 in assets. Most states have exercised the option to target Medicaid Home and Community-Based waiver services to those whose incomes are less than 300 percent of SSI income limit, or $19,872 per year in 2004 (O'Keeffe and Wiener, 2004, see also Kassner and Shirley, 2000).

Although the eligibility standards differ, there is substantial overlap between the people who are eligible to be served under Medicaid and the various housing programs. Using income data from the 2000 March Current Population Survey and matching it to the local AMI limits established by HUD, the Lewin Group found that all people aged 65 and older who met the basic SSI level of eligibility were also eligible for housing subsidies at 50 percent of the AMI. Since the SSI level is much lower than housing eligibility limits, only 11 percent of those eligible for housing subsidies met the SSI level of eligibility for Medicaid. The programs are better matched at the 300 percent of SSI criteria commonly used for eligibility under Medicaid waiver programs. Roughly three-fourths (76 percent) of older persons who met the 300 percent of SSI income level were also eligible for housing subsidies at 50 percent of the AMI, and 95 percent of those who were eligible for housing subsidies would also be eligible for Medicaid waiver services (Commission on Affordable Housing, 2002).

Table 14 estimates the percentages of older homeowners and renters who may be eligible for Medicaid or at risk of being eligible by virtue of their low incomes and levels of disability.[8] The table estimates Medicaid risk by using the 300 percent of SSI income level and the disability measure of difficulty with bathing, dressing, and getting around the house, a rough proxy for risk of nursing home admission.[9] Using these measures, one out of six older residents in subsidized housing (16.5 percent) are at heightened risk of Medicaid eligibility, compared to one out of 12 renters without subsidies (8.8 percent) and one out of 20 homeowners (5.0 percent).

Table 15 shows the percentage of those at heightened risk of Medicaid eligibility by virtue of their low incomes and levels of disability who are owners, renters without subsidies, and renters with subsidies. Although renters who receive subsidies constitute only 4.9 percent of all persons aged 65 and older, they represent 13.2 percent of all persons who are at heightened risk of Medicaid eligibility. Indeed, about one-third of all older persons at heightened risk of Medicaid eligibility are renters, which suggests that strategies to target services might extend beyond subsidized housing to market rate rental housing with large concentrations of older persons with low incomes.

TABLE 14. Percentage of Persons Aged 65 and Older with Various Housing Tenures by Risk Factors for Medicaid Eligibility

	Income < 300% SSI	Income < 300% SSI + Difficulty Bathing, Dressing, and Getting Around the Home
Owners	43.9	5.0
Renters, No Subsidy	62.4	8.8
Renters, With Subsidies	91.2	16.5
Total	48.7	6.1

Source: 2002 American Communities Survey, Analysis by AARP PPI staff.

TABLE 15. Percentage of Persons Aged 65 and Older with Various Risk Factors for Medicaid by Housing Tenure

	Owners	Renters, No Subsidy	Renters, With Subsidies
Total, All Incomes	81.7	13.3	4.9
Income < 300% SSI	73.8	17.1	9.1
Income < 300% SSI + Difficulty Bathing, Dressing, Getting Around the Home	67.5	19.2	13.2

Source: 2002 American Communities Survey, Analysis by AARP PPI staff.

These estimates of Medicaid risk are rough approximations that are intended to give a picture of the relative risks experienced by older renters in subsidized housing compared to those in other types of housing. The American Communities Survey does not collect data on assets, but the data from Table 13 suggest that if an asset limit were included renters with subsidies would have constituted a much higher percentage of those at risk of Medicaid eligibility. Perhaps more importantly, these estimates focus on Medicaid eligibility criteria and do not incorporate the additional risk factors such as marital status, informal supports, and race. In short, housing subsidy programs have very efficiently, if inadvertently, targeted a population at high risk of needing supportive services to manage their disabilities and of needing Medicaid to pay for these services.

THE CAPACITY OF HOUSING PROGRAMS TO DELIVER SERVICES

The congregate living arrangements for older persons in subsidized housing projects and the risk profile of the residents in those projects would seem to offer a unique opportunity to target services in a way that may prevent or delay costly nursing home services among those most at risk. But providing services that achieve the goal of promoting independence for these residents depends on the capacity of the housing settings to provide such services. The capacity to deliver supportive services in subsidized housing projects varies enormously, depending on both the physical characteristics of the housing complex and the sponsor's experience with service provision.

Housing Characteristics

Due to limitations in the data sources, this article has reported data on all renters with subsidies whether or not they live in projects especially built to meet the needs of older persons though many of those renters live in mixed age communities that are not likely to be targets for linking housing and services programs for older persons. Research conducted for the Commission on Affordable Housing and Health Facility Needs for Seniors in the 21st Century (2002) indicates that roughly 800,000 apartments are in projects specifically built to serve older persons.[10] Because of the economies of scale, targeting services to these projects may be the most efficient way to link housing and services.[11]

Projects built to serve older persons also have the advantage of including many accessibility features and common spaces that are essential to serve residents with disabilities. The availability of key features varies by type of housing: Section 202 projects for the elderly, Low Income Housing Tax Credit (LIHTC) projects built for older persons, and mixed age LIHTC projects (see Table 16).

By virtue of their physical make-up, some housing facilities are more capable of providing supportive services than others. Larger facilities with commercial kitchens, dining areas, and other common spaces may be able to add services with relatively little retrofitting. Smaller facilities with limited common spaces may be ill equipped to provide such services without having to make major alterations. Unfortunately, as federal funding for building new housing that meets the needs of older persons declined in recent years, more smaller facilities with fewer amenities have been built. Moreover, cost-containment measures instituted in the mid-1980s severely limited common spaces for services. More than 60 percent of Section 202 facilities occupied before 1984 provided congregate dining compared to half (29 percent) of those projects occupied in the mid-1980s (Heumann, Winter-Nelson, and Anderson, 2001).

Sponsors of projects serving older persons that decide to add an assisted living level of services face an additional set of challenges adapting their physical plants (Wilden and Redfoot, 2002). Even when they include accessibility features and common spaces, subsidized housing projects are rarely designed in an optimal way to offer assisted living services. For example, security features that are necessary to serve persons with dementia are generally missing, and few facilities meet the building codes and other regulatory requirements associated with licensure for assisted living. Early experience with HUD's Assisted Living Conversion program indicates that adding such features can be difficult and expensive, though the demand for these services is large (Hilton, 2004). In some cases, housing sponsors have built adjoining assisted living fa-

TABLE 16. Percentage of Section 202 and Low Income Tax Credit Housing Projects Serving Older Persons with Various Supportive Features

	Section 202 (1999)	LIHTC Projects for Older Persons (2001)	LIHTC Mixed Age Projects (2001)
Grab Rails	73.9	60.3	17.5
Ramps or Level Entry	91.1	91.4	57.9
Emergency Phone Number	80.1	83.7	60.8
Common Meeting Room	90.2	86.0	22.8

Sources: Heumann, Winter-Nelson, and Anderson, 2001; Kochera, 2002.

cilities rather than attempt costly and disruptive retrofitting (Wilden and Redfoot, 2002).

The Service Component

The number of subsidized housing projects providing intensive services is growing but remains a small fraction of all projects. Undoubtedly the biggest improvement in the capacity of housing projects to serve older persons with disabilities has been the addition of service coordinators on staff. Until the housing acts of 1990 (42 U.S.C. 8012)[12] and 1992 (12 U.S.C. 1701(q)(g)[13] HUD would not allow housing sponsors to include any social services staff in their budget requests except for the few projects participating in the CHSP. Since the authorization and subsequent funding of service coordinators in fiscal year 1993, the number of service coordinators has grown dramatically. The 1999 National Survey of Section 202 found that 37.4 percent of elderly housing projects now have service coordinators on staff (Heumann, Winter-Nelson, and Anderson, 2001). A 2001 survey found that 21 percent of housing projects for older persons funded by the Low Income Housing Tax Credit program had a service coordinator on staff and another 47 percent indicated that service coordination was available in the community (Kochera, 2002).[14] Although comparable survey data do not exist on other housing programs, a 1998 report estimated that 3,700 resident service coordinators were employed in federally subsidized housing nationwide (Mokkler and Monks, 1998).

Having service coordinators on staff does not in itself allow projects to offer intensive on-site service programs, but coordinators are able to connect residents with many supportive services that allow them to remain independent. The 1998 report on service coordinators found that the services most frequently used by their clients were housekeeping (85.0 percent), home health care (83.7 percent), and personal care assistance (79.0 percent) (Mokkler and Monks, 1998). In a HUD evaluation, coordinators agreed that the program was effective in "improving the quality of life for the residents, linking residents with the services they need to continue living independently, and assessing and monitoring residents' needs for and use of services" (Department of Housing and Urban Development, 1996b).

Services provided by housing staff have generally focused on those services that benefit the whole community rather than targeting services to those most at risk. For example, both the Section 202 and LIHTC survey found that the most commonly provided services by far were social and recreational (Heumann, Winter-Nelson, and Anderson, 2001; Kochera, 2002). To the extent that services require additional capacity from the building, staff-provided services may be declining, especially in newly constructed buildings. In general, the 1999 survey of Section 202 housing found that older projects were far more likely to offer supportive services than newer projects, which may reflect the larger size and greater physical capacity of the older projects. Fifty-nine percent of projects occupied before 1974 offered meals or housekeeping services compared to less than 20 percent built since the mid-80s (Heumann, Winter-Nelson, and Anderson, 2001). Only 23 percent of all Section 202 projects (Heumann, Winter-Nelson, and Anderson, 2001) and 16 percent of housing facilities for older persons financed by the LIHTC program provided group meals (Kochera, 2002).

On the other hand, services from providers other than housing staff appear to be increasing, perhaps in part because service coordinators are helping renters to receive services from outside providers. Table 17 shows the relative growth of staff-provided services and services provided by outside providers in Section 202 projects built before 1988. Staff-provided services show modest increases, but services from other providers show substantial increases.

As discussed earlier, a small, but important program that successfully links services to housing subsidized renters with disabilities has been the federal CHSP. Enacted in 1978, the CHSP funds congregate services in approximately 100 subsidized housing projects. Most funds go toward service coordination and meals; however, the CHSP has been effective in leveraging other supportive services such as housekeeping, transportation, and personal care (U.S. House of Representatives, 1987).

In addition to laying the foundation for the service coordinator program, the federal CHSP has also served as a model for a number of state programs. The state and federal CHSP programs have provided the basis in some states for expanding services still further to include assisted living in subsidized housing. For example, New Hampshire expanded its federally funded CHSP program to housing authorities throughout the state, using Medicaid waivers to

TABLE 17. Percentage of Residents Receiving Services in 1999 and 1988 from Facility Staff and Other Providers in Section 202 Projects Existing in 1988[15]

	Facility Staff		Other Providers	
	1988	1999	1988	1999
Personal Care	0.8	1.7	7.7	19.6
Housekeeping	2.1	4.4	15.6	26.4
Transportation	4.1	6.2	19.1	33.1

Source: Heumann, Winter-Nelson, and Anderson, 2001.

provide health-related services beyond the basic CHSP model in subsidized housing projects (Martin and Salloway, 1997).

Several states have gone still further to provide assisted living services in subsidized housing. New Jersey has the most extensive program of this type, using its statewide CHSP as a base for expanding to assisted living services. The state developed a new licensing category specifically to encourage assisted living programs in subsidized housing projects (Crystal, Kurland, and Rosenthal, 1996). Fourteen service providers are currently licensed to provide assisted living programs in 37 different subsidized housing projects. New Jersey uses Medicaid waivers to provide support for both the CHSP and assisted living programs and is seeking state funding for residents who are not eligible for Medicaid.

Similarly, Maine now includes its CHSP as one of three "assisted living" licensure categories–along with adult family care homes and residential care facilities. The state's Bureau of Elder and Adult Services characterizes congregate housing services as "Maine's preferred type of assisted living" because the regulations require private apartments with individual bathroom and food preparation areas. More than 300 individuals are served by congregate "assisted living" (State of Maine, 2001).

Despite these efforts, only a small minority of subsidized housing projects provides the intensive level of services needed by residents at high risk of nursing home admission. The LIHTC survey found that only two percent of projects for older persons were licensed as assisted living or residential care facilities (Kochera, 2002). Using a definition of providing 24-hour on-site supervision, homemaker services, and personal care services, the 1999 Section 202 survey identified 5.1 percent of projects as assisted living, though the survey did not ask how many were licensed to provide assisted living services (Heumann et al., 2001).

OVERCOMING OBSTACLES
TO LINKING HOUSING AND SERVICES:
POLICY IMPLICATIONS

The network of federally subsidized housing has enormous potential to promote the independence of older persons with disabilities by linking housing with supportive services. The characteristics of older residents in subsidized housing described in this article indicate a high level of need for such services. The significant risk of needing Medicaid assistance to pay for supportive services, especially the high cost of nursing home services, should provide the incentive for public policymakers to promote supportive housing alternatives. This final section will identify policy issues that must be resolved before subsidized housing can realize its potential to serve older persons with disabilities. (See Pynoos, Liebig, Alley, and Nishita, 2004, in this volume for a more extensive discussion of policy issues related to linking housing and services.)

1. Services programs and housing programs must work together to take advantage of the efficiencies that such housing may offer in providing supportive services to residents at high risk.

Housing programs may have efficiently targeted those at high risk, and housing projects may offer the economies of scale associated with offering home- and community-based services (HCBS) to a number of people at one site, but housing and services programs are not structured to take advantage of those efficiencies (see O'Keeffe and Wiener, 2004, in this volume for a more extensive discussion of Medicaid and housing). The article noted some of the differences in eligibility criteria in Section II, but those differences are trivial compared to the basic differences in approaches to providing and financing services.

Housing programs require large commitments of capital over a long period of time, typically 15 to 30 years. Unfortunately, public and private sources of capital have paid too little attention to how the buildings they finance must adapt to the changing needs of their renters as they age in place over time. For example, the Low Income Housing Tax Credit program forbids the financing of "healthcare facilities," which has inhibited the provision of nursing and other health-related services. Section 202 facilities have become smaller over time with fewer facilities needed to provide services.

Subsidized housing projects are unlikely to build new facilities, undertake major capital improvements, or hire staff related to providing services in the absence of funding commitments for those services. At the same time, services programs, especially state Medicaid programs, have generally not been willing or able to make long-term commitments to provide services in specific housing projects. Without long-term commitments to funding services in a housing project, housing sponsors are often unwilling to take the risks associated with building or converting to affordable assisted living.

Linking housing and service provision is not simple, but examples from the Coming Home program (described in greater detail in another article in this issue, Jenkens et al., 2004) demonstrate that it can be done. An essential aspect of this Robert Wood Johnson Foundation-funded demonstration was its requirement that housing, finance, social services, and healthcare agencies work together. Beyond the affordable assisted living projects already built, the Coming Home program aims to leave a lasting legacy by altering state systems and forging interagency relationships.

2. Housing programs will require a significant infusion of capital to retool for the new mission of serving older persons with disabilities.

According to the American Communities Survey over 1.8 million people aged 62 and older are served by housing subsidy programs, which is more than the number of older people who are in nursing homes. The provision of these subsidies has required a significant commitment of capital over the past 50 years. Preserving that housing stock and retrofitting existing buildings to serve the growing number of older renters with disabilities will require a new round of investment from public and private sources. Early experiences with the Section 202 conversion program suggest that funding should be flexible enough to allow for the construction of new units as well as the retrofitting of existing units. The oldest projects may be the best candidates for such investments for several reasons (Wilden and Redfoot, 2002):

- the oldest projects house the oldest and most disabled residents;
- retrofitting could be done in conjunction with general modernization needed by older buildings;
- older projects in both Section 202 and public housing are more likely to have large numbers of efficiency units, which are difficult to market as regular housing but may be more suitable for affordable assisted living; and,
- older projects are generally larger and are more likely to have kitchens and dining areas.

Questions remain over how much money should be spent on new construction versus on preserving and retrofitting current housing. Another more philosophical question is the degree to which housing programs should target scarce resources on serving older renters with disabilities. When subsidized housing units are in short supply, enabling one person with disabilities to age in place longer means denying a unit to someone on the waiting list. The Seniors Housing Commission projects that the demand for subsidized housing for older persons will escalate, but that housing production will not increase as rapidly as demand (Commission on Affordable Housing, 2002).

3. All levels of government have to be committed to successfully link housing and services, but the primary locus for decision-making should be with the state agencies responsible for providing and regulating supportive services.

Although federal resources are needed and local commitment is essential, the most successful efforts in providing service-enriched housing on a broad scale have resulted from concerted multi-agency initiatives by the states.[16] States have the primary responsibility for policy decisions affecting LTC services. States administer the Medicaid program, even though most of the money comes from the federal government, and they regulate the types of services offered. Although HUD programs are administered by the federal agency, Low Income Housing Tax Credits are administered by state housing finance agencies.

One way to target federal resources to support state supportive housing initiatives could be to increase funding to the CHSP. The CHSP is authorized to give grants to states as well as to individual projects, which allowed two states (New Hampshire and Connecticut) to develop impressive supportive housing programs throughout their states. One feature of the CHSP that was never implemented was dubbed "Project Retrofit" by its congressional authors. Project Retrofit was intended to supply grants for capital improvements that would allow housing projects to provide supportive services. A competitive grant program like CHSP, which has the flexibility to fund capital costs and limited services, could provide the incentive for states to be more active partners in planning and overseeing the conversion to service-enriched housing. Making states the applicants might also avoid some of the problems faced by the Assisted Living Conversion program, where matching requirements for funds and licensure requirements have been stumblingblocks for projects wanting to participate.

4. Committing funds for housing and services must be matched by a commitment to enhance the quality of care and the quality of life experienced by older renters with disabilities.

Much of the renewed interest in linking housing and services for older persons with disabilities has been motivated by a desire to save money. Rapidly escalating Medicaid costs have generated a flurry of activity among states looking for low costs alternatives to nursing home care, but demonstrating savings by offering alternative home- and community-based services has been difficult.[17] Targeting services to rente rs in subsidized housing may offer one of the most cost-effective interventions, but providing high quality services will not be inexpensive. It would not be a worthy public policy goal to replicate the experience of the mental health field by allowing subsidized housing projects to become poor quality, underfunded board and care facilities serving a highly disabled, deinstitutionalized population.

Offering service-enriched housing is best thought of as a part of a more comprehensive approach to reforming LTC financing and service delivery (AARP, Public Policy Institute, 2003). Comprehensive reform should fund an array of housing and service options to meet the varied needs and preferences of older persons with disabilities. Halfway measures that simply add a few poorly funded alternatives are not likely to save money or provide quality services to those who need them.

States that have made a commitment to systematic reforms have found that they can decrease the number of older persons in nursing homes while offering greater consumer choice and quality service. These states may also save some money (Alecxih et al., 1996), but more importantly they have shown that it is possible to serve more people with disabilities in settings that they prefer without breaking the bank. The data presented in this article suggest that linking supportive services with subsidized housing can play an important role in a comprehensive strategy to enhance the quality of LTC services as well as the privacy, dignity, and autonomy of older persons with disabilities.

NOTES

1. This estimate comes from the 2002 American Communities Survey (ACS). The estimate corresponds closely to Kochera's 2001 estimate of 1.7 million older households served by federal housing programs.

2. The ACS is a large nationwide survey conducted by the Census Bureau to collect information on persons and households. Because it is part of the Census Bureau's strategy to re-engineer the 2010 Census, most of the content is identical to the long form of the 2000 Census. However, a few variables have been introduced that did not appear on the 2000 Census long form, including information on the presence of a rental subsidy. In 2003, the ACS included information from approximately 1 million persons living in 460,000 households.

3. The Survey of Income and Program Participation is a nationwide survey conducted by the Census Bureau to collect information about income, demographics and participation in public programs. The survey is designed around a core panel, with subsequent interviews over a period of about three years. The panel for 2001 includes 36,700 households, interviewed nine times from February 2001 through January 2004. During the course of the interviews, supplemental information is periodically collected about household wealth.

4. Owners of housing projects for older persons financed by the Low Income Housing Tax Credit program estimated that 34 percent of their residents were frail in a 2001 survey (Kochera, 2002).

5. The 1999 survey of Section 202 housing found a very similar ratio of women to men—77.6 percent women to 22.4 percent men (Heumann, Winter-Nelson, and Anderson, 2001).

6. The ACS does not directly collect information on the categories used in this table. Instead, the ACS collects open responses regarding "ancestry or ethnic origin." Racial categories (e.g., White, Black, Asian), as well as ethnic origin (e.g., Hispanic), were assigned by Census personnel based on the October 30, 1997 Federal Register Notice entitled, "Revisions to the Standards for the Classification of Federal Data on Race and Ethnicity," issued by the Office of Management and Budget (OMB). It is pos-

sible for a single individual to have more than one race, and the ethnic category of "Spanish/Hispanic/Latino" was assigned separately from race.

7. The 50 percent of AMI limit for a single person ranges from $12,800 in rural Mississippi to $39,600 in San Francisco. Some older projects subsidized by HUD set income levels at 80 percent of AMI. Low Income Housing Tax Credit projects generally have an income limit of 60 percent of AMI.

8. The American Communities Survey does not include information on assets, one of the factors used to qualify for SSI. The analysis here proxies for SSI eligibility solely on the basis of income. In 2002, the federal SSI level was $545 for individuals and $817 for couples. Tables 14 and 15 use 300 percent of those numbers, since most state Medicaid programs use that standard for HCBS waivers. The disability measure used here asks, "Because of a physical, mental, or emotional condition lasting six months or more, does this person have any difficulty in doing any of the following activities . . . Dressing, bathing, or getting around in the home?" We used this measure because it most closely corresponds to ADL limitations and because it appears to measure the highest level of disability among the measures used by the American Communities Survey (see Table 4).

9. O'Keeffe (1996) found that states vary enormously in the health and disability criteria they use to determine nursing home eligibility under Medicaid. In general, most states include medical criteria that exceed the disability measure used in this study.

10. If these apartments serve roughly the proportion of married couples indicated by Table 8, it would suggest that between 900,000 and 1,000,000 individuals are living in subsidized projects for older persons.

11. HUD conducted a small demonstration, HOPE for Elderly Independence, with 16 public housing projects to link services and housing vouchers for subsidized renters not living in projects for older persons. The program had difficulty locating people who qualified at the high level of disability required under the program. But those served appeared to benefit from the combination of service coordination, personal care, and housekeeping offered under the program (Department of Housing and Urban Development, 1996a).

12. 42 USC 8012 amended the National Housing Act of 1959 to allow service coordinators in Section 202 housing.

13. 12 USC 1701(q)(g) added authority for service coordinators in other public and assisted housing serving older persons or persons with disabilities.

14. Service coordinators in LIHTC projects are not generally funded by HUD but must come from the operating budgets of the projects. The survey of tax credit projects did not identify the source of funding, the number of hours worked, or the qualifications of the service coordinators.

15. The 1999 Section 202 survey included both external agencies and family and friends in the "Other Provider" category in order to make it compatible with the 1988 survey (Heumann, Winter-Nelson, and Anderson, 2001).

16. For more thorough discussions of what states have done and could do to develop linkages between housing and services see Pynoos et al. (2004), Jenkens et al. (2004), Sheehan and Oakes (2004), and Tillery (2004) in this volume of the *Journal of Housing for the Elderly*.

17. For a discussion of the research on potential cost savings from home and community-based services, especially as it applies to services in subsidized housing, see Golant (2003).

REFERENCES

AARP Public Policy Institute. (2003). *Beyond 50.03: A Report to the Nation on Independent Living and Disability.* Washington, DC: AARP.

Alecxih, Lisa Marie B., Steven Lutzky, John Corea, and Barbara Coleman. (1996). *Estimating Cost Savings from the Use of Home and Community-Based Alternatives to Nursing Home Care in Three States.* AARP Public Policy Institute Publication No. 9618. Washington, DC: AARP.

American Communities Survey. (2002). U.S. Census Bureau; generated by Andrew Kochera, AARP Public Policy Institute; using public use microdata <http://www. census. gov/acs/www/Products/PUMS/pums2002.htm> (30 March 2004).

Bishop, Christine E. (1999). "Where Are the Missing Elders? The Decline in Nursing Home Use, 1985 and 1995." *Health Affairs,* Vol. 18, No. 4, July/August, pp. 146-155.

Black, Betty Smith, Peter V. Rabins, and Pearl S. German. (1999). "Predictors of Nursing Home Placement Among Elderly Public Housing Residents." *The Gerontologist,* Vol. 39, no. 5, pp. 559-568.

Commission on Affordable Housing and Health Facility Needs for Seniors in the 21st Century (Seniors Commission). (2002). Report to Congress, Washington, DC.

Crystal, Stephen, Carol H. Kurland, and Lila Rosenthal. (1996). *Expanded Services for Frail Elderly Tenants.* New Brunswick, NJ: Rutgers University, Institute for Health, Health Care Policy, and Aging Research.

Damon-Rodriguez, J., S.P. Wallace, and R. Kington. (1994). "Service Utilization and Minority Elderly: Appropriateness, Accessibility and Acceptability." *Gerontology & Geriatrics Education,* Vol. 15, pp. 45-64.

Department of Housing and Urban Development. (1999). *Housing Our Elders: A Report Card on the Housing Conditions and Needs of Older Americans.* Washington, DC: U.S. Department of Housing and Urban Development.

Department of Housing and Urban Development. (1996a). *Evaluation of the HOPE for Elderly Independence Demonstration Program: Second Interim Report.* HUD Report No. 1616-PDR. Washington, DC: U.S. Department of Housing and Urban Development.

Department of Housing and Urban Development. (1996b). *Evaluation of the Service Coordinator Program.* HUD Report No. 1613-PDR. Washington, DC: U.S. Department of Housing and Urban Development.

Department of Housing and Urban Development. (1995). *American Housing Survey.* 1995. Washington, DC: U.S. Department of Housing and Urban Development.

Dilworth-Anderson, Peggye, Ishan Canty Williams, and Brent E. Gibson. (2002). "Issues of Race, Ethnicity, and Culture in Caregiving Research: A 20-Year Review (1980-2000)." *The Gerontologist,* Vol. 42, No. 2, pp. 237-272.

Golant, Stephen M. (2003). "Political and Organizational Barriers to Satisfying Low-Income U.S. Seniors' Need for Affordable Rental Housing with Supportive Services." *Journal of Aging & Social Policy,* Vol. 15, No. 4, pp. 21-48.

Golant, Stephen M. (1999). *The CASERA Project: Creating Affordable and Supportive Elder Renter Accommodations.* Gainesville: University of Florida.

Hawes, Catherine, Charles D. Phillips, and Miriam Rose. (2000). *High Service or High Privacy Assisted Living Facilities, Their Residents, and Staff: Results for a National Survey.* U.S. Department of Health and Human Services, Office of the Assistant Secretary for Policy and Evaluation. Washington, DC.

Heumann, Leonard, Karen Winter-Nelson, and James Anderson. (2001). *The 1999 National Survey of Section 202 Housing for the Elderly.* AARP Public Policy Report #2001-02. Washington, DC: AARP.

Hilton, Lisette. (2004). "Making Affordable Assisted Living Viable." *Practices.* March/ April, pp. 34-37.

Himes, Christine L., Dennis P. Hogan, and David J. Eggebeen. (1996). "Living Arrangements of Minority Elders." *Journal of Gerontology,* Vol. 51B, No. 1, pp. S42-S48.

Jenkens, Robert, Paula C. Carder, and Lindsay Maher. (2004). "The Coming Home Program: Creating a Road Map for Affordable Assisted Living Policy, Programs, and Demonstrations." *Journal of Housing for the Elderly,* Vol. 18, No. 3/4, pp. 179-201.

Kassner, Enid, and Lee Shirley. (2000). *Medicaid Financial Eligibility for Older People: State Variations in Access to Home and Community-Based Waiver and Nursing Home Services.* Washington, DC: AARP.

Kochera, Andrew. (2001). "A Summary of Federal Rental Housing Programs." *Public Policy Institute Fact Sheet # 85.* Washington, DC: AARP.

Kochera, Andrew. (2002). *Serving the Affordable Housing Needs of Older Low-Income Renters: A Survey of Low-Income Housing Tax Credit Properties.* AARP Public Policy Institute Report No. 2002-7. Washington, DC: AARP.

Martin, Tamara A. and Jeffrey Salloway. (1997). *Evaluation, The Tavern Alternative Housing Program: Providing Alternative Housing for Low-Income Seniors.* Concord, NH: The New Hampshire Health Care Transition Program.

Mokkler, Pamela M., and Janice C. Monks. (1998). "National Resident Service Coordinators' Perceptions Study: The Role of Service Coordination in Independent Housing Communities." *Quality Aging Solutions Report.*

National Center for Health Statistics. (2002). *The National Nursing Home Survey: 1999 Summary.* Washington, DC: U.S. Department of Health and Human Resources, National Center for Health Statistics.

National Long-Term Care Survey, 1999. (2003). U.S. Census Bureau data, initial analyses done for AARP's Public Policy Institute by the Urban Institute, Washington, DC.

O'Keeffe, Janet and Joshua Wiener. (2004). "Public Funding for Long-Term Services for Older People in Residential Care Settings." *Journal of Housing for the Elderly,* Vol. 18, No. 3/4, pp. 51-79.

O'Keeffe, Janet. (1996). *Determining the Need for Long-Term Care Services: An Analysis of Health and Functional Eligibility Criteria in Medicaid Home and Community-Based Waiver Programs.* AARP Public Policy Institute Report #9617. Washington, DC: AARP.

Pynoos, Jon, Phoebe Liebig, Dawn Alley, and Christy M. Nishita. (2004). "Homes of Choice: Towards More Effective Linkages Between Housing and Services," *Journal of Housing for the Elderly,* Vol. 18, No. 3/4, pp. 5-49.

Redfoot, Donald L. and Sheel M. Pandya. (2002). *Before the Boom: Trends in Long-Term Supportive Services for Older Americans with Disabilities.* AARP Public Policy Institute Report No. 2002-15. Washington, DC: AARP.

Sheehan, Nancy W. and Claudia E. Oakes. (2004). "Public Policy Initiatives Addressing Supportive Housing: The Experience of Connecticut," *Journal of Housing for the Elderly,* Vol. 18, No. 3/4, pp. 81-113.

Spector, William D., John A. Fleishman, Liliana E. Pezzin, and Brenda C. Spillman. (2000). *The Characteristics of Long-Term Care Users.* Publication No. 00-0049. Rockville, MD: Agency for Healthcare Policy and Research.

State of Maine, Bureau of Elder and Adult Services. (2001). "Overview of Maine's Assisted Living Programs." Presented at the "Coming Home" program sponsored by the Robert Wood Johnson Foundation and the National Cooperative Bank.

Stone, Robyn. (2000). *Long-Term Care for the Elderly with Disabilities: Current Policy, Emerging Trends, and Implications for the Twenty-First Century.* New York: Milbank Memorial Fund.

Stucki, Barbara, and Janemarie Mulvey. (2000). *Can Aging Baby Boomers Avoid the Nursing Home?* Washington, DC: American Council on Life Insurance.

Survey of Income and Program Participation. (1996). U.S. Census Bureau, 1996 panel, wave 12 (approximately Q1 2000); generated by Andrew Kochera, AARP Public Policy Institute; using public use microdata downloaded via "Data Ferrett"; <http http://www.sipp.census.gov/sipp/access.html>; (30 March 2004).

Tillery, Debra. (2004). "Supportive Housing Initiatives in Arkansas." *Journal of Housing for the Elderly,* Vol. 18, No. 3/4, pp. 115-136.

U.S. House Select Committee on Aging. (1987). *Dignity, Independence, and Cost-Effectiveness: The Success of the Congregate Housing Services Program.* House Report No. 100-650.

U.S. Senate Special Committee on Aging. (1975). *Congregate Housing for Older Adults: Assisted Residential Living Combining Shelter and Services.* Senate Report No. 94-478.

Wallace, Steven P., Lene Levy-Storms, Raynard S. Kington, and Ronald A. Anderson. (1998). "The Persistence of Race and Ethnicity in the Use of Long-Term Care." *Journal of Gerontology,* Vol. 53B, No. 2, pp. S104-S112.

Wilden, Robert and Donald L. Redfoot. (2002). *Adding Assisted Living Services to Subsidized Housing: Serving Frail Older Persons with Low Incomes.* AARP Public Policy Institute Report #2002-01, Washington, DC: AARP.

STATUTES CITED

42 U.S.C. 8012
12 U.S.C. 1701(q)(g)
Public Law 95-557, The Congregate Housing Services Act of 1978

Assisted Living for Lower-Income and Frail Older Persons from the Housing and Built Environment Perspective

Leonard F. Heumann

SUMMARY. This paper examines the linkages between housing and supportive services from the built environmental perspective. When it comes to linking supportive services, it is usually true that the wealthier an individual is the more private resources he or she has available to define a personal support system at every step in the aging process; the poorer the individual is, the fewer choices she or he has and the successful linkages of government subsidized housing, health and supportive services become more important to successful aging of that person. Low-income and aging individuals are the real testing ground for whether current policy allows holistic support linkages to occur and whether programs are available in both the quantity and quality to empower low-income older persons with options and support choices.

The discussion that follows is limited to supportive services and aging in place in conventional housing and affordable purpose built assisted living programs and facilities; it omits institutional living. For low-income older persons, institutional care provides few if any housing choices or individual power to control support delivery, and thus

---

[Haworth co-indexing entry note]: "Assisted Living for Lower-Income and Frail Older Persons from the Housing and Built Environment Perspective." Heumann, Leonard F. Co-published simultaneously in *Journal of Housing for the Elderly* (The Haworth Press, Inc.) Vol. 18, No. 3/4, 2004, pp. 165-178; and: *Linking Housing and Services for Older Adults: Obstacles, Options, and Opportunities* (eds: Jon Pynoos, Penny Hollander Feldman, and Joann Ahrens) The Haworth Press, Inc., 2004, pp. 165-178. Single or multiple copies of this article are available for a fee from The Haworth Document Delivery Service [1-800- HAWORTH, 9:00 a.m. - 5:00 p.m. (EST). E-mail address: docdelivery@haworthpress.com].

linkages between cooperating support professionals and programs becomes increasingly moot. *[Article copies available for a fee from The Haworth Document Delivery Service: 1-800-HAWORTH. E-mail address: <docdelivery@haworthpress.com> Website: <http://www.HaworthPress.com> © 2004 by The Haworth Press, Inc. All rights reserved.]*

KEYWORDS. Long-term care, housing, aging, affordable, public policy, Medicaid, low-income, subsidized housing, assisted living, built environment

BACKGROUND TRENDS

There are three trends to keep in mind before examining the quality of assisted living programs for lower-income Americans. First, society is aging and the need for supportive services is growing (Commission, 2002). Second, the older low-income population is the most likely to find the cost of assisted living out of reach. Third, the subsidized housing stock of assisted living as well as the presence of community-based supports when living in conventional housing is under-supplied (Heumann, Winter-Nelson, and Anderson, 2001; Kochera, 2002).

Two years ago, the Second World Assembly on Aging sponsored by the United Nations in Madrid reported that at current trends the population aged 60 and over will triple to two billion people in the next 50 years (Associated Press, 2002). In the United States and other developed countries the associated economic crisis caused by aging trends will come more rapidly due to gains in longevity and the shrinking proportion of working taxpayers to retirees. Alan Greenspan, the Federal Reserve chairman, recently made a dire prediction of the costs of these aging trends on American taxpayers. Although his solution of trimming Social Security benefits is being called into question, there is no doubt that this year's record $521 billion deficit will, as he reported, get worse once 77 million baby boomers become Social Security eligible in just four years. Furthermore, the benefits promised under Medicare could create an even larger deficit based on what the current program promises and the probability of costly medical advances in coming years (Crutsinger, 2004).

In the housing arena there is a growing crisis in what lower-income seniors can afford in the way of assisted living services. A recent Fannie Mae Foundation report on "Making Affordable Assisted Living a Reality" concluded that this crisis is looming because the average annual fee for housing and services in assisted living is $32,400 per year, while 64% of older persons have annual incomes under $25,000 (Schuetz, 2003).

The supply of affordable rental housing with and without supportive services is actually dwindling relative to the growing demand among older persons. The building of new public housing exclusively for older persons has stopped. At the same time much of the "family" public housing–including where "young" older persons are raising grandchildren–is being torn down. New construction Section 8 senior housing projects have been halted, and much of the existing stock is at-risk of conversion to market rate units or is already converted. This leaves only the Section 202 and the Low Income Housing Tax Credit (LIHTC) programs, both of which are severely under-funded in the current federal and state tight budget economies (as described further below).

The LIHTC, unlike Section 202, is not exclusively for older low-income persons; only about 80% of these properties are developed entirely for low-income persons, and only 24% are intended primarily for older persons (Kochera, 2002). In order to provide truly affordable housing and assisted living services for older low-income residents, both programs still need Project Rental Assistance Contracts or tenant based rental assistance through housing vouchers or certificates, as well as waivers for home- and community-based service (HCBS) or other grants and subsidies. Only the most recent phase of the Section 202 program has the option to provide subsidized assisted living services. The vast majority of existing Section 202 and LIHTC properties for older persons can only provide supportive and assisted living if the property owners can find additional funds and manage to overcome the differences in requirements and monitoring between funding sources, which are daunting tasks. Both the legislation and the regulations of the two existing programs fail to fully address the need for funding supportive services for aging resident populations (Heumann, Winter-Nelson, and Anderson, 2001; Kochera, 2002).

The next three sections of this paper provide a more in-depth look at the Section 202 program, the LIHTC program, and HCBS programs from a housing perspective. The goal is to determine if these three programs provide a comprehensive package of support and adequate choices to meet the lifestyle needs of the wide variety of low-income older persons who will be aging in place in the coming years.

THE SECTION 202 HOUSING PROGRAM

Under the Section 202 program, local non-profit organizations including churches, synagogues, mosques, labor unions, and fraternal organizations can apply for federal funding to own and manage a senior housing facility, of which over 3,500 existed nationwide in 1998. There have been three national surveys of the Section 202 program (U.S. Senate, 1984; Gayda and Heumann,

1989; Heumann, Winter-Nelson, and Anderson, 2001). The surveys were completed by both the owners/sponsors of the facilities and the site managers. The 2001 report concluded that typical Section 202 facilities provide secure, affordable and barrier free environments by caring staff that, to varying abilities, are attempting to adapt their facilities' environments and support services to the needs of their aging residents. At the same time, the findings of both the 1989 and 2001 reports showed that the Section 202 program was not keeping pace with the demand for this type of housing and some phases of the program could not adequately support aging in place.

The Section 202 program has been subject to five changes in policy and design over the years and each phase has had different effects on the program's ability to provide affordable assisted living. The Moderate-Income phase (1959-74) had the highest income eligibility requirement with generally no rental assistance and had the largest facilities (148 units on average). The Low-Income phase (1974-84) had Section 8 rental assistance serving renters with less than 80% of median income (89 units on average). The Cost-Containment or Very Low-Income phase (1985-88) served renters below 50% of median income and had small facilities (54 units on average). Facilities in this phase were built under rigid cost cutting rules that limited common space and other amenities needed for aging in place. The Transition phase (1989-94) waived the cost-containment measures but continued with the lowest-income eligibility rules and smaller facility size (52 units per facility on average). Financing varied depending on the timing of the project between the previous and subsequent PRAC phase (1993-present), which uses "project rental assistance contracts" instead of Section 8 rental assistance. Eligibility and smaller unit size (50 units on average) remain the same as in the two previous phases, but the PRAC phase has well built facilities and encourages care management and support assistance with daily living.

The existing Section 202 population is aging in place whether or not affordable assisted living is provided. The average age has been rising steadily from 72 in 1983, to 73.6 in 1988, to 75 in 1999. Simple extrapolation puts the average age between 76 and 77 in 2004. The managers reported 13.0% of residents to be frail in 1988; this rose to 22.3% in 1999. Financial support is the primary reason people apply to a Section 202 facility; however, the older and frailer the resident the more the managers report that supportive services, improved security, and increased social contacts are important.

Overall, 37.4% of Section 202 facilities had an on-site staff service coordinator in 1999, 43.8% relied on community-based service coordination, and 18.7% had no service coordinators to help frail residents. In 1999 site managers at facilities with service coordinators reported that service coordinators increased the range of supportive services (90.5% of respondents), increased the quality of services (78.3%), and allowed residents to stay independent longer (81.1%). Provision of on-site congregate services such as meals and house-keeping increased between 1988 and 1999 only for facilities built in the earliest two program phases. Over 58% of the Moderate Income phase facilities reported on-site congregate services in 1999, compared to 38% in the Low-Income phase and 12.9%, 10.5%, and 18.7% in the three most recent phases. Some of this variation is explained by a higher proportion of residents aged 80 and over considered frail by the managers of the older facilities. It also reflects that the two earliest phases are more likely to have facilities with residents who can afford to pay for these services, financial reserves that can be used to subsidize these costs, and common space to accommodate communal kitchens, common dining, and space for on-site housekeeping staff.

The survey results show that it has been getting more difficult to care for the frailer residents. The single most dramatic change from 1988 to 1999 was site management complaints about hospitals releasing residents too soon. These complaints rose from 26.7% in 1988 to 77.5% in 1999 and might reflect the impact of the implementation of the Medicare Prospective Payment System. In addition, the percentage of managers reporting that their facilities were not set up to handle applicants with critical support needs actually increased from 1988 to 1999, primarily due to the newer phases of the program being unable to handle such cases (13.4% in 1999).

The single most troubling statistic reported in 1988 and 1999 was that new Section 202 construction *was not* keeping up with the demand for affordable housing units in the growing and aging low-income population. Nationwide, the waiting time was eight years in 1988 and nine years in 1999. On average, there were nine older persons waiting for every 202 unit that became vacant in 1999. In large cities, which have high concentrations of older persons, the waiting time in 1999 was eleven years.

On the positive side, an increasing number of Section 202 facilities are providing some assisted living services. Many facilities have their own on-site staff and programs, but the most common way they access services is through community-based programs. Facilities built in the two earliest phases and the PRAC phase often either have tenants who are able to pay for services or access to funding reserves or special subsidized programs that enable them to retrofit their facilities to accommodate congregate services and still keep rents and support costs affordable. On the negative side, Section 202 facilities built during the Cost-Containment and early Transition phases are particularly ill equipped to provide any support. Their residents have the lowest income eligibility requirements, they have no financial reserves, and the facilities have little or no common space for congregate dining and socializing. For the most part these facilities lack both scale-economies and room to retrofit and provide supportive services. In fact, there has been a decrease in full-time site management at these facilities and higher numbers of managers reporting that they lack the capabilities to accept more frail applicants.

Finally, there are signs that the average Section 202 facility is finding it harder to retain aging and frail residents even as the demand for Section 202 housing is higher than ever and new construction is lagging far behind demand. Most people who inquire about a unit probably never even apply due to the extremely long waiting list. The obvious and urgent recommendations that stem from these observations are: (1) the construction of more new Section 202 facilities; (2) the funding of more retrofitting of existing facilities to accommodate aging in place; and, (3) the provision of more comprehensive subsidized supportive services.

THE LOW-INCOME HOUSING TAX CREDIT PROGRAM

The Low-Income Housing Tax Credit (LIHTC) provides tax credits or earned income shelters to qualified housing providers who can then sell these credits to limited partners to raise funds to construct or rehabilitate housing. In return, 20 to 40 percent of the units must be set aside for low-income residents at affordable rents. Unlike the Section 202 program, which is a federal budget line-item program, the LIHTC program is funded by allotting tax credits that reduce individual income tax payments. In addition, the LIHTC program is run by state housing agencies that are allotted a pool of tax credits by the federal government. The goals of the program are to both involve what is hoped will be more efficient private-for-profit developers in the subsidized housing market and to provide properties that house a mix of renters by income and avoid concentrating low-income residents in specific projects. For-profit developers often partner with nonprofit sponsors/managers to provide this affordable housing.

The LIHTC program has become the major federal subsidized housing program for building and rehabilitating affordable housing, yet relatively little research has been conducted on the people housed by the program and how effective (or ineffective) the program is in terms of meeting residents' needs. This is particularly true for properties that house predominantly older low-income residents. The data in this section comes from an AARP report on a national survey of LIHTC properties (Kochera, 2002), the only such study to date. It is based on 1,558 survey returns from 10,000 randomly selected mailed questionnaires sent to property owners in 2001.

The LIHTC is currently funding 70,000 new affordable rental units annually, more than 15,000 of which are "designated primarily for older persons." This makes LIHTC projects the largest subsidized housing source for older persons given that Section 202 produces fewer than 10,000 new units each year. A cautionary note is required, however, because "designated primarily for older persons" simply means that ". . . the owner indicated (the property) was intended for older persons and more than half the resident households included at least one person aged 62 or older" (Kochera, 2002, p. v).

Similar to Section 202 facilities, LIHTCs designated for older persons have extremely low vacancy rates (a national average of just 3%). The average waiting period for an available unit is eight months. This is not as severe as the nine year waiting time for Section 202 units, but the study shows that tax credit properties for older persons are more often located in suburbs and rural areas than in central cities, and tend to be small facilities with an average of only 32 units. The Section 202 data showed that waiting time was higher in larger cities where more of the older low-income population is concentrated. Many LIHTC projects tend to be built in low-density service areas where the most common additional subsidy program has been Department of Agriculture Rural Housing Services below-market interest rate mortgages.

One-third of the LIHTC facilities for older persons had no access to a service coordinator compared to 18.7% for Section 202 housing. As in most Section 202 housing, service coordination is usually provided by community-based agencies (47%), as are congregate services (e.g., meals or housekeeping service). The availability of full or partial congregate services was about the same in tax credit and Section 202 facilities (e.g., group meals 16% in LIHTC versus 14% in Section 202; housekeeping 13% in LIHTC versus 19% in Section 202). Tax credit properties with at least one nonprofit sponsor were far more likely to offer supportive services than properties sponsored exclusively by for-profits. In other words, tax credit properties for older persons that had a Section 202 management profile were more supportive of aging in place.

The conclusions of the Kochera study are quite troubling. First, the tax credit units for older persons are going primarily to suburbs and rural areas, even though older low-income persons are concentrated in the largest cities. Second, although larger properties tend to have economies of scale that make the provision of services more likely and more affordable to low-income residents, the average size of LIHTC properties is too small (32 units) to provide service scale economies. Third, community-based services are less plentiful and have larger and therefore costlier areas to cover in low-density suburbs and rural areas. Fourth, the legislation and funding regulations for the LIHTC program fails to address the needs of affordable supportive services that help older residents successfully age in place. When owners/sponsors consider applying for other subsidy grants or programs to provide affordable supportive services, they encounter discouraging requirements, monitoring criteria, and procedures that make it difficult or impossible to provide the combination of subsidized housing and services. Finally, similar to the Section 202 program, the demand or need for affordable LIHTC units far outweighs the supply.

Supportive Housing Conclusions

It is very unlikely in the current political and tight budget climate that the states or the federal government will either resurrect the public housing program or legislate and fund any new subsidized housing programs for older persons. Despite the many common problems and shortcomings, both the LIHTC and Section 202 programs seem to provide excellent affordable housing facilities and have sensitive sponsors/managers that have the desire but not the funding streams to assist their frail and aging low-income residents to age in place. Neither program alone can provide the variety of housing, supportive services, and locations needed by the diverse low-income aging population, but together they present a variety of choices. The for-profit development and the combination of for- and nonprofit owners under the LIHTC program produces a variety of important alternatives to the predominantly religious-based non-profit Section 202 housing. The differences in the owner/manager types have already resulted in different site locations that provide older persons meaningful location options. The differences in facility sizes should also result in another form of lifestyle choice for applicants, and this size variety can be enhanced if adaptations in the two program policies can be coordinated to form a comprehensive affordable housing package in the future. The different management agents that are likely chosen by tax credit ventures and religious-based Section 202s should also provide important choice options. The fact that the tax credit facilities are not restricted to very low-income eligibility (as in Section 202 facilities) allows them to provide a mix of incomes among older residents and, thus, to create a different type of social setting and lifestyle choice.

In fact, the combination of these two established and apparently effective affordable housing alternatives presents the potential for excellent variety in housing type, management, and location choices. The key, of course, remains being able to set aside enough tax credit units and enough funding for both new construction and retrofitting of existing Section 202 units so that both programs are large enough to give realistic options to older low-income applicants in every local market. It also means funding adequate amounts of supportive services to allow management to help residents age in place in both programs and do so in ways that monitor for excellence and efficiency without destroying variety and flexibility in support delivery.

DEFINING HOLISTIC COMMUNITY BASED ASSISTED LIVING

Older persons continually express a desire to age in their own homes for as long as possible (AARP, 2000). This has helped spur the growth and popularity of HCBS, which provide aging and frail residents assistance with various ADLs and IADLs in their own homes. The growing popularity has extended HCBS from conventional housing to subsidized housing, where subsidized versions of these programs have become particularly important in extending the lives of low-income frail older persons. As was shown in both of the latest surveys of Section 202 and LIHTC housing, managers of properties under both programs rely more often on HCBS vendors than in-house staff.

Research over the years has identified various examples of HCBS for older persons in subsidized and conventional housing in developed countries (Heumann and Boldy, 1983; Heumann and Boldy, 1993; Heumann, 1997; and Heumann, McCall, and Boldy, 2001). Research has shown that such programs can efficiently serve low-income older persons, keep them relatively independent in their own homes, and actually postpone or eliminate the need to move to purpose built assisted living or institutional care. In addition, the development of case management has made the delivery of HCBS more holistic while also simplifying, personalizing, and dignifying the process. The tremendous pressure to measure efficient use of HCBS by showing high ratios of older persons served, however, has caused older low-income persons located in areas that are dangerous (e.g., with high crime rates) or sparsely populated (e.g., fringe suburbs and rural locations) to be underserved. Even if they receive HCBS, low-income consumers in such areas often only receive the "economy version," meaning they have no choice of vendors, no weekend or evening services, and only the most basic elements of needed support.

Traditional HCBS programs are designed, and their funding streams are often limited to, human service provision and its management. There is at least one set of services that is frequently missing from HCBS programs; these programs are often not designed to incorporate universal design features and management into their service models.

A study of HCBS programs in Melbourne illustrated that absence of the environmental component (Heumann, 1997a; 1997b). The study consisted of site visits and interviews with 23 coordinators of care. The study analyzed a variety of program characteristics by type, range of care services, risk of over-caring or under-caring, and cost-effectiveness. Imbedded among the interview questions were three that specifically addressed housing and environmental adaptations as part of a holistic care service.

The Melbourne study found that all coordinators indicated that twelve specified services were provided by the programs: care management, meals, homemakers, personal care, nurses, physical and occupational therapy, respite, recreation, transportation, podiatry, and hair care. Laundry, religious ministries, personal budgeting and financial counseling, speech pathology, psychiatric visits, and extended holiday programs were mentioned by one or more coordinators when asked in an open-ended question what additional services were provided. No one mentioned repair, adaptations, or additions to the physical housing unit or the use of new physical devices to aide frail and disabled clients.

When asked directly about services such as home maintenance, modifications, or new physical devices, 18.2% of the coordinators said that they had a full range of such services available because their programs were run out of a hospital, nursing home, homeless shelter, or other facility with a maintenance staff that could make home repairs or modifications. Another 45.5% said that they had a partial solution, such as a city service that they could call on as long as costs remained low and the staff was used sparingly. Finally, 36.4% of coordinators said that their care managers just did not or could not deal with any aspect of the built environment.

In the final question the coordinators were presented with a statement that there might be too much emphasis on client assessments that measure physical and mental support needs provided by formal and informal caregivers and not enough evaluation of the client's physical environment and how it can be adapted. The statement continued with: "By not assessing the barriers in the home and not adapting the environment or providing mechanical devices, we failed to let the client do more for themselves on their own."

There were three groups of responses to this statement: only 18.2% said that environmental solutions were provided and were a vital part of their care management model; 27.3% agreed with the statement saying that their management model focused on visiting human services and not enough on environmental solutions; finally, 54.3% disagreed in part or whole with the statement. Some liked the idea of being able to provide more environmental adaptations, but not the mechanical or electrical devices that they considered cost prohibitive or something their clients would find alien and reject. Some understood the need to focus on environmental solutions but noted that reimbursement streams prevented it. Others interpreted the statement as attempting to totally eliminate human services and said that would be a mistake because so many of their clients were isolated and relied on visiting services for the psychological benefits.

Experience has demonstrated that when outside funds and extra planning resources are available, care managers in British, American and Australian HCBS programs have ramps built and grab-bars installed in the bathrooms of very disabled persons' homes. It is much rarer to see service managers with traditional HCBS resources who are capable or willing to provide comprehensive environmental assessments that result in changes such as user friendly door handles, window openings or a safer and easier to use lighting (Pynoos, Tabbarah, Angelelli, and Demiere, 1998). In many cases, they cannot even provide something as basic as a washer and dryer. Instead they assign a homemaker to take a client's laundry to a Laundromat and sit for 2 1/2 hours/week at $18.00/hour, costing the program over $2,000/year when for under $1,000 a washer and dryer could be provided in the client's unit, used for several years, and then reused by other clients in the future. The visiting human support system is so segregated from built environment solutions that such support is totally overlooked.

If human service solutions are the only way to address support needs of frail older persons, it is questionable if older persons are actually being empowered and given lifestyle choices to deal with their aging related disabilities, and it is questionable if traditional HCBS is truly holistic and cost-efficient. All 23 of the Melbourne coordinators defined their mission as keeping older persons in their private homes with the highest level and quality of life possible and all felt they were succeeding with well managed, cost-efficient and caring programs. They all had ways to monitor over- or under-caring, but most were at least partially ignorant of how to assess and modify the built environment (or they lacked the funding capability to do so).

THE DEVELOPMENT
OF A COMPREHENSIVE CARE MANAGEMENT SYSTEM

HCBS in the United States play a pivotal role in assisted living for older low-income persons whether they live in conventional housing or in subsidized purpose-built housing for older persons. Typical HCBS programs, however, are not designed to incorporate universal design options and management into their service models. Their focus is on human support service delivery, as is their funding stream and the training of their professional care managers. Only older persons who know to solicit the right assistance and can privately afford it can put together *truly comprehensive* care management that assesses their capabilities and their environment holistically. Even then, it is rare that an individual can obtain truly comprehensive care management through one universally trained advocate.

Universally trained advocates need broad-based training. With the early release of recuperating patients from hospitals due to current HMO and insurance practices, older persons require knowledgeable *medical case management* when they return to the community. They also need *social service case management* to understand the wide array of visiting support options and to orchestrate care delivery that minimizes invasive visits on personal privacy, adjusts to the changing client needs and tastes, and continues to maximize independence. In addition, older persons need *environmental care assessment, repair and renovation management.* This is the most frequently absent care management skill and service, yet the lower the income the more substandard the environment (in both the home and the surrounding neighborhood) is likely to be, and the more important the environmental management becomes to retaining maximum independence.

In short, a new holistic care manager is needed who has public health, social work, housing, and neighborhood planning skills. The more frail and dependent a person is, the more vital it is to receive a holistic package of care management skills and services in order to maximize his/her quality of life and ability to live independently.

COORDINATED HOUSING, PUBLIC HEALTH
AND SOCIAL SERVICES

There are a number of broader implications to achieving comprehensive and coordinated assisted living. First, it is important to emphasize that more affordable housing options are needed along with a larger supply of housing for frail older persons in advance of the baby boomers' retirement. Second, more holistic management and increased subsidies are needed so that a full array of affordable support vendors can be accessed. In addition to combining all the pertinent professional fields in gerontology to develop holistic and affordable policy and programs, a new comprehensive care coordination curriculum needs to be developed for professional graduate schools to produce care managers who are truly capable of assessing and managing the combined health, social services and environmental support needs of frail older persons.

Finally, a support system needs to be developed that encourages older persons to remain active and knowledgeable participants in all their decisions so that they can be their own best planners and advocates. True empowerment of older persons is the key to cost containment and affordable support. Older persons who remain as independent and knowledgeable as possible about their housing and support options will ultimately provide cost savings. An educated and informed consumer is the key to an effective, democratic free-market LTC system.

Policymakers need to be conscious of the micro-neighborhood environments and ensure that they provide the widest variety of choice for that culture. This level of holistic planning might be best suited to a "neighborhood planner-gerontologist and community advocate"–another new professional type to accommodate a diverse and growing aging population. These neighborhood planners are envisioned as people who can position themselves to represent health, social service and environmental infrastructures as needed and who are not bound to any one of these service fiefdoms. Flexibility will be the key to enable all supportive living components to be integrated into the flow of society.

REFERENCES

AARP. (2000) *Fixing to Stay: A National Survey on Housing and Home Modifications Issues*, Washington, D.C., AARP.

Associated Press. (2002) Conference to Focus on Graying of Humanity (Madrid, Spain), Washington, D.C., *Champaign, News Gazette*, April 3, 2002, pp. A-1 and A-10.

Commission on Affordable Housing and Health Facility Needs for Older Persons in the 21st Century. (2002) *A Quiet Crisis in America*, Washington, D.C., Commission on Affordable Housing and Health Facility Needs for Older Persons in the 21st Century.

Crutsinger, Martin. (2004) Greenspan Urges Social Security Cuts. Washington, D.C., *Associated Press*, March 26, 2004.

Gayda, Kathy S. and Leonard F. Heumann. (1989) *The 1988 National Survey of Section 202 Housing for the Elderly and Handicapped*, Washington, D.C., Subcommittee on Housing and Consumer Interests of the Select Committee on Aging, House of Representatives, December 1, 1989, USGPO, Comm. Pub. No. 101-736.

Heumann, Leonard F. (1997a) Aging in Conventional Housing: A Planner's Evaluation of the New Australian Home Based Care Management Programs, Part 1, *Australian Planner*, Volume 34, Number 1, pp. 143-48.

Heumann, Leonard F. (1997b) Aging in Conventional Housing: A Planner's Evaluation of the New Australian Home Based Care Management Programs, Part 2, *Australian Planner*, Volume 34, Number 2, pp. 189-94.

Heumann, Leonard F. (Ed.). (1997) *Managing Care, Risk and Responsibility: The Challenge of the 21st Century as the Aging and Disabled Population Grows and Diversifies*, The Proceedings, SYSTED 97, Champaign, IL: University of Illinois Press.

Heumann, Leonard F. and Duncan Boldy (Eds.). (1993) *Aging in Place with Dignity: International Solutions to Accommodate the Low Income and Frail Elderly*, Westport, CT: Praeger Books.

Heumann, Leonard F. and Duncan Boldy. (1983) *Housing for the Elderly: Planning and Policy Formulation in Western Europe and North America*, London, Croom Helm, New York: St. Martins Press.

Heumann, Leonard F., Mary McCall and Duncan P. Boldy (Eds.). (2001) *Empowering Frail Elderly People: Opportunities and Impediments in Housing, Health and Support Service Delivery*. Westport, CT: Greenwood Publishing Group.

Heumann, Leonard F., Karen Winter-Nelson and James R. Anderson. (2001) *The 1999 National Survey of Section 202 Elderly Housing*, Washington, D.C., Public Policy Institute, AARP, Report # 2001-02, 106 pp.

Kochera, Andrew. (2002) *Serving the Affordable Housing Needs of Older Low-Income Renters: A Survey of Low-Income Housing Tax Credit Properties*, Washington, D.C., Public Policy Institute, AARP, Report #2002-07, 98 pp.

Pynoos, Jon, Melissa Tabbarah, Joe Angelelli, and Marian Demiere. (1998). Improving the Delivery of Home Modifications. *Technology and Disability*. Vol. 8. pp. 3-14.

Schuetz, Jenny. (2003) Making Affordable Assisted Living a Reality, *Housing Facts & Findings*, Fannie Mae Foundation, Washington, D.C., Vol. 5, No. 3 pp. 1, 4-7.

U.S. Senate, Special Committee on Aging. (1984) *Section 202 Housing for the Elderly and Handicapped: A National Survey*, Washington, D.C.: U.S. Government Printing Office.

The Coming Home Program:
Creating a State Road Map
for Affordable Assisted Living Policy,
Programs, and Demonstrations

Robert Jenkens
Paula C. Carder
Lindsay Maher

SUMMARY. This paper describes barriers and opportunities to creating affordable assisted living facilities for older persons eligible for Medicaid services. This information is based on the practical experiences of the Coming Home Program, a project of NCB Development Corporation (NCBDC) with funding from the Robert Wood Johnson Foundation (RWJF). Begun in 1992, this national program has contributed to the creation and adoption of state policies including regulations, implementation of state programs, creation of development and operational feasibility analysis tools, and the identification and structuring of financing sources. It has also fostered and supported public-private partnerships that have resulted in 31 operational affordable assisted living demonstration projects with another 73 in development.

[Haworth co-indexing entry note]: "The Coming Home Program: Creating a State Road Map for Affordable Assisted Living Policy, Programs, and Demonstrations." Jenkens, Robert, Paula C. Carder, and Lindsay Maher. Co-published simultaneously in *Journal of Housing for the Elderly* (The Haworth Press, Inc.) Vol. 18, No. 3/4, 2004, pp. 179-201; and: *Linking Housing and Services for Older Adults: Obstacles, Options, and Opportunities* (eds: Jon Pynoos, Penny Hollander Feldman, and Joann Ahrens) The Haworth Press, Inc., 2004, pp. 179-201. Single or multiple copies of this article are available for a fee from The Haworth Document Delivery Service [1-800- HAWORTH, 9:00 a.m. - 5:00 p.m. (EST). E-mail address: docdelivery@haworthpress.com].

The paper explains the need for affordable assisted living, Coming Home's definition of affordable assisted living, and the structure of the Coming Home Program. Four case studies are presented that summarize the goals and outcomes of the Coming Home Programs in Arkansas, Florida, Washington, and Vermont. The paper's conclusions provide lessons learned during the program's first twelve years and their implication for state policies and programs. *[Article copies available for a fee from The Haworth Document Delivery Service: 1-800-HAWORTH. E-mail address: <docdelivery@haworthpress.com> Website: <http://www.HaworthPress.com> © 2004 by The Haworth Press, Inc. All rights reserved.]*

KEYWORDS. Long-term care, housing, aging, affordable, assisted living, Medicaid

THE NEED FOR AFFORDABLE ASSISTED LIVING

Assisted living is the fastest growing private-pay long-term care (LTC) model in the United States. It is clearly the preferred LTC option for upper-income persons when they can no longer remain at home. Unfortunately, it is typically not an option for persons with low-incomes. Nationally, the average annual cost of assisted living is $28,548 a year (MetLife, 2003), yet 47% of Americans aged 65 and older have annual incomes of less than $25,000. Of the 10.2 million households of people aged 75 years and older, the group most likely to need LTC services, 65% percent have incomes under this amount.

The need for assisted living in rural communities and for low-income populations has been increasing for many years, as indicated by the recent report, "A Quiet Crisis in America," compiled by the Commission on Affordable Housing and Health Facility Needs for Seniors in the 21st Century (2003). Rural communities have a higher percentage of older persons than urban areas (15% compared to 12%), and older persons living in rural communities have limited access to community-based alternatives. In addition, poverty levels are often high for older persons living in rural areas. In 1998 over half of non-urban persons aged 85 and older were classified as poor or near poor, with incomes at 100% to 149% of the poverty level. Over half of households headed by a person aged 85 or older reported annual incomes of less than $10,000 (Rogers, 1999).

Unfortunately for the almost 35% of Americans aged 65 and older who will need Medicaid subsidies if they require LTC, states still limit the majority of their Medicaid funding to nursing home care. Where Medicaid is available for assisted living, the programs often have long waiting lists or do not pay enough to purchase acceptable quality services from private market providers.

To make high quality assisted living available to persons with low-incomes, state Medicaid programs must provide sufficient funding for assisted living subsidy programs, and states must foster the development of programs focused on serving Medicaid eligible individuals.

THE COMING HOME PROGRAM'S DEFINITION OF AFFORDABLE ASSISTED LIVING

State and provider definitions of assisted living vary widely. Perceptions of what is affordable are also subjective. The Coming Home Program is interested in developing high quality models of assisted living that are similar to the best practice models available for private market consumers and that can be available to Medicaid eligible residents as a nursing home alternative. As such, Coming Home defines assisted living as a program that implements assisted living's values of maximizing consumer control, independence, and dignity by providing:

- resident-directed assessment and care planning;
- 24-hour awake staff sufficient to meet the scheduled and unscheduled needs of very frail and cognitively impaired tenants;
- full services programs including care planning, personal care, medications management and administration, meals, housekeeping, laundry, and coordination of transportation and programs to meet psychosocial needs;
- private occupancy, accessible apartments; and,
- sufficient common and service space.

The Coming Home Program definition of assisted living excludes providers who offer only "light care" programs intended as a pre-nursing home service.

NCBDC defines an "affordable" project as one that makes 25% or more of its units and services available to persons using Medicaid to pay for services and SSI-level incomes to pay for rent and meals.

THE COMING HOME PROGRAM

The Coming Home Program was created to address the needs of older persons who required affordable supportive housing, especially in rural and low-income areas. In the late 1980s, RWJF funded the development of two assisted living demonstration projects in rural North Carolina as part of an initiative to coordinate LTC services with existing acute care health providers. NCBDC, a non-profit organization providing lending and technical assistance to projects serving disadvantaged communities, had a long history of financing affordable housing and health care clinics in economically distressed areas.

Phase I: Demonstrating the Viability of Affordable Assisted Living Facilities

To explore solutions for premature institutionalization and lack of access to affordable community-based services, RWJF provided a grant to NCBDC in 1992. The program goal included identifying and selecting a small number of rural communities and local organizations to create models of affordable assisted living. As the National Program Office, NCBDC provided pre-development loans and intensive technical assistance to selected projects. The technical assistance included feasibility, development and operational consulting. NCBDC also facilitated partnerships between the projects and state agencies to craft demonstration programs where necessary, and to overcome regulatory obstacles, policy conflicts, and subsidy gaps in state housing and service programs.

From 1992 to 1997, these Phase I demonstration projects and their partners identified successful strategies to deliver high quality, high service assisted living programs that fully encompassed the values of privacy, dignity, and autonomy. Alongside these strategies, the Coming Home Program identified the state policy and program elements necessary to support these strategies and the long-term stable operations of affordable assisted living.

Phase I resulted in the construction of five affordable assisted living projects in four states.[1] These projects attracted approximately $22 million in grants, tax credits, and mortgages and led to the creation of an effective template for affordable assisted living financing, service delivery, and architectural design.

The First Coming Home Demonstration

A good example of a Phase I demonstration project is Cache Valley Assisted Living Apartments (Cache Valley), located in a rural area of Southern Illinois. When Cache Valley was built in 1993 there were no low-income elderly rental apartments in the area, and the few nursing homes all had lengthy waiting lists. People aged 65 and over comprised 18% of the total population of this area (which had 45,984 people in total) at that time. The region had the highest unemployment and poverty rates in Illinois, and income levels among the lowest in the country. In 1992, 77% of older persons in this region had annual incomes below $15,000.

Cache Valley has 40 apartments. Each resident has a private, accessible apartment with a kitchenette and full bath. All residents meet the state nursing home medical eligibility criteria. By combining several development subsidy programs (e.g., low-income housing tax credits and HOME, the grant program established by the Home Investment Partnership Act of 1990) with a small amount of conventional debt, the initial rents at Cache Valley were reduced to between $300 and $400 a month. A Medicaid pilot project covered the service costs for eligible residents. Combining real estate subsidies and Medicaid made the project 100% affordable to individuals at 60% of the local area median income.

Lessons Learned in Phase I

Making affordable assisted living a reality in Cache Valley and the other demonstration sites revealed a host of policy and programmatic obstacles that prevent developers and sponsors from pursuing affordable assisted living projects. The conflict between housing subsidy and licensing requirements (e.g., low-income housing tax credit program prohibitions against frequent or continual nursing services), the mismatch between annual service subsidy appropriations and lenders' long-term capital commitment, and the need to obtain multiple funding sources to finance a project all discourage organizations from attempting to develop affordable assisted living.

Although there were several committed individuals and organizations at each site, none had the expertise to combine housing and health service programs. Phase I revealed that technical expertise, knowledge transfer, and policy work are essential to success and replication. In southern Illinois, this has proven to be the case. Cache Valley's sponsoring organization has continued to develop additional assisted living projects for itself as well as assisting other organizations in that area.

Phase II: Working with State Governments to Encourage Further Development

The Phase I demonstration projects proved that public agencies, service providers, non-profit groups, and community advocates were interested in creating affordable assisted living to serve Medicaid-eligible individuals and that they could partner effectively to overcome difficult policy and financial barriers. Phase II built on these lessons, and the Coming Home Program is currently working with nine state governments to create the environment and supports required to foster development of affordable assisted living resources. The program continues to serve as a catalyst and capacity building mechanism for the demonstration programs. These efforts, in turn, serve as models for other states interested in increasing the supply of affordable alternatives to institutional care.

Phase II began in 1998 and is scheduled to end in 2005. This phase is structured to provide grant support and technical assistance to state governments and to create a policy environment that supports the development and operation of affordable assisted living. In order to receive the grants, states committed to:

1. analyze obstacles and gaps in their regulatory, service, and housing programs;
2. implement the policy and program elements and reforms necessary to address the identified gaps and obstacles; and,
3. recruit and assist organizations to develop affordable assisted living projects to demonstrate their viability in the state's new environment.

NCBDC provides coordinated grant support, technical assistance, and loan funds to help states create a policy environment that supports affordable models of assisted living targeted to Medicaid-eligible individuals. In addition, NCBDC and state grantees establish partnerships with existing community health care systems, non-profit housing and social service groups, and community-based organizations to develop affordable demonstrations.

Grant Awards

The first stage in Phase II included awarding grants to qualified states. NCBDC, working with RWJF and a National Advisory Committee, awarded grants of up to $300,000 to nine states[2] over a three-year period. The criteria for the state applicants included:

1. the application had to come from one of three state agencies (the unit that administers the assisted living program, the Medicaid office, or the housing finance agency) and had to include a commitment from each agency to work together to solve the policy and program barriers identified under the grant;
2. the state had to have in place or be ready to implement a reimbursement mechanism to fund the services for Medicaid-eligibles aged 65 and older;
3. the state Housing Finance Authority had to include older adults as a priority group;
4. the partner agencies had to form a state advisory committee comprised of consumers, providers, state agencies, and other stakeholders to identify barriers to developing and operating affordable assisted living projects serving Medicaid-eligible individuals;

5. the proposed activities had to have the potential to create systemic change in state financing and regulatory systems to encourage the development of affordable assisted living;
6. the proposal had to include recruitment and support for demonstration projects; and,
7. the states were required to provide a cash or in-kind match for each year of the program.

Demonstration Project Criteria

The state project officers disseminate information on the Coming Home Program and recruit demonstration projects. The selection criteria include:

1. locating a non-profit sponsor in good standing;
2. providing a minimum of 25% of their units to Medicaid-eligible individuals;
3. committing to the high service levels required by Medicaid-eligible residents, including licensing under the state's assisted living category; and,
4. providing accessible private occupancy apartments, including kitchenettes and full bathrooms.

Pre-Development Loan Fund

Phase II continues to provide demonstration projects access to an $8 million pre-development loan fund created jointly by RWJF and NCBDC and administered by NCBDC. The loan fund provides capital for non-profit sponsors of affordable assisted living and may be used to pay for:

1. feasibility and market studies;
2. project consultants, including developers, architects, engineers, and operations consultants;
3. site control; and,
4. studies required for design, financing, or local approvals.

Eligibility for the loans is restricted to projects that:

1. are located in a Coming Home State;
2. are approved by the state Coming Home project director;
3. provide a minimum of 25% matching support, including a minimum of $10,000 in a cash match; and,
4. are acceptable to NCBDC under the underwriting criteria established for the demonstrations.

The loans cannot exceed $100,000 and may not be used for staff salaries or fund raising. A variety of limits apply to how much of the loan funds may be used for various activities. Interest accumulates at 6% per year and loans are for a maximum of two years. Loans are repaid at the end of two years or at construction funding, whichever occurs first.

The loans provide critical access to high risk capital for organizations that have a mission to provide affordable assisted living but do not have the capital to risk exploring an unfamiliar and complex project. The pre-development loan provides these organizations with unsecured debt at a low cost in order to pursue feasibility and development work. The loans allow the Coming Home Program to share the risk of exploring project viability with local organizations. A cash match is required to provide evidence of strong organizational commitment to the project–a critical requirement as the projects often navigate significant obstacles throughout their two to three year development process.

Technical Assistance

The Coming Home Program continues to provide ongoing, intensive technical assistance to the grantee states and demonstration projects, including:

1. *performing policy analyses* (e.g., working with the state's Medicaid agency and the grant's advisory committee to identify obstacles and create solutions, including implementation of or modifications to a state's home and community-based services (HCBS) waiver program or regulations);
2. *performing financial analysis* (e.g., working with non-profit social service and medical care providers to create viable development and operations *proformas* and to identify and access required public and private funds for services and housing);
3. *providing development assistance*, including consulting on development and operating analyses, market studies, and identification of development team (architects, engineers, specialty consultants for financing and subsidy applications, and contractors); and,
4. *facilitating communication* among the various stakeholders, including community providers, state agencies, and financing sources.

In addition, NCBDC has created tools to support development and policy activities including a state policy manual, a feasibility analysis program, and documentation and links to emerging best practices in affordable assisted living.

STATE CASE STUDIES

This section chronicles the development of four affordable assisted living programs in four states. Though a large number of organizations and individuals participated in the creation of policies, financing, and development of affordable assisted living facilities under the Coming Home Program, these four state case studies were chosen to represent different approaches, regulatory mandates, and partnerships. The information for the case studies comes from annual reports provided to the Coming Home Program, materials collected for presentations at national and regional conferences, and conversations with the Coming Home Program officers and demonstration sponsors in each state (see Table 1).

Each state case study includes the overall needs and goals identified for the state program, the partnerships, initial challenges, demonstration project development process, and state lessons.

Arkansas Coming Home Program

Needs and Goals. Arkansas has the seventh highest percentage of persons aged 65 and older in the U.S. In 1995, the state ranked 14th in the nation for total poverty, but had the highest percent of persons aged 65 and over living in poverty. Nearly half of Arkansans aged 65 and older have an annual income of less than $20,000. According to the Arkansas Office of Long-term Care, in 2002 more than 23,000 Arkansans with chronic medical needs required services in a residential facility with most of them living in a nursing facility.

TABLE 1. Four States and Demonstration Project Examples

| State | Demonstration Project | | | | |
	Name	Location	Project Financing	Number of Units	% Affordable Assisted Living
Arkansas	The Gardens at Osage Terrace	Bentonville	• Low-income housing tax credits (LIHTC) • HOME • Federal Home Loan Bank Affordable Housing Program	45	100%
Florida	Helen Piloneo Assisted Living Facility	Pinellas	• Bond issue by public housing authority	110	100%
Vermont	Cathedral Square Assisted Living	Burlington	• HUD Assisted Living Conversion Program grant	28	75%
Washington	Quail Hollow	Chewelah	• U.S. Department of Agriculture Rural Development Program	16	50%

At the date of the state's application for the Coming Home Program award (2000), Arkansas did not have regulations defining assisted living or a Medicaid waiver (1915c) covering assisted living services although the state agencies were committed to and had already begun creating both.

Partnerships. The Arkansas Department of Human Services Division of Aging and Adult Services partnered with the Office of Long-Term Care and the Arkansas Development Finance Authority to apply for the grant. The Arkansas Department of Human Services Division of Aging and Adult Services received the Coming Home grant.

Initial Challenges and Successes. In order to meet the goals, the state had to take the following four important steps:

1. The Department of Human Services had to develop draft regulations for assisted living. This two-year process was affected by vested interests from other LTC providers and health professionals accustomed to nursing home standards who were concerned about the perceived safety and quality limitations presented by assisted living.
2. The State Health Service Commission had to develop a Permit of Approval Process for assisted living facilities. The administrators of Mercy Health Systems were hesitant to contract as service providers until it was certain that the state would adopt regulations and the permit process.
3. In order to create an affordable alternative to nursing facilities, the State Department of Human Services planned to apply for the Medicaid HCBS waiver 1915(c) and, thus, the ultimate reimbursement rate was uncertain.
4. In order to ensure that the rental portion of assisted living fees would be affordable, the state had to make a variety of public grant and financing sources available. The State Finance Development Authority committed to creating a LIHTC set aside for affordable assisted living facilities that met program requirements, in addition to designating a percentage of its HOME program allocation.

Demonstration Project. The Arkansas Department of Human Services Division of Aging and Adult services and NCBDC worked with the Community Development Corporation of Bentonville/Bella Vista, Inc. (CDC) to foster the development of The Gardens at Osage Terrace (The Gardens). The Gardens is a 45-unit affordable assisted living project. The service and rent charges for all 45 units are affordable to individuals with incomes as low as $564 per month (the Federal SSI payment amount in 2004). The Gardens utilizes Medicaid and real estate subsidy programs to provide this level of affordability.

Although an experienced housing developer, the CDC was not a service provider. The CDC partnered with Mercy Health Systems of Northwest Arkansas, Inc. (Mercy), a local, mission driven hospital to provide the assisted living services at The Gardens. The CDC, as the facility owner, manages the building (e.g., leasing, rent collection, and maintenance) and accepts any net income or loss associated with the real estate. Mercy provides the services (e.g., staffing, assessments, care and meal delivery, services billing), maintains the assisted living license, and receives any net income from services. Mercy also accepts full responsibility for any loss associated with the services.

When the CDC started development of The Gardens, the state was in the process of drafting regulations for assisted living and applying for a Medicaid waiver to fund assisted living services. The CDC mitigated the risk posed by the evolving policy process in three ways. First, the CDC participated in the state's development process for the new assisted living regulations, ensuring a strong voice for affordable assisted living needs in the formulation of the regulations. Second, the CDC designed the facility to comply with or exceed the anticipated physical requirements contemplated for the regulations (only slight modifications were required in The Garden's plans after the regulations were completed). Finally, they established a viable alternative, or "Plan B," to operate The Gardens as an independent living residence with in-home care if an assisted living development became impossible for regulatory or financial reasons.

Five programs were utilized to finance The Gardens, including the Coming Home Program's pre-development loan, LIHTC, a private mortgage, a Federal Home Loan Bank Affordable Housing Program (FHLB AHP) grant, and a HOME loan. In addition, they received a grant from the Community Care Foundation. The LIHTCs accounted for 57% of the total development cost. The LIHTC program provides equity to projects by providing a grant of tax credits that a non-profit organization can sell to investors to offset the investors tax liability. The LIHTC, HOME, and AHP programs each have significant rules and requirements governing resident eligibility, design, and operational considerations. The ability to underwrite the project as affordable assisted living with independent housing as an alternative provided lenders and investors the assurance they needed to finance the project. The CDC's choice of an experienced service partner with a shared mission and financial depth was also critical to building confidence in the project.

While The Gardens is structured to accept persons with incomes as low as the federal SSI amount ($564 in 2004), the real estate subsidies programs used allow The Gardens to rent to individuals at or below 60% of the area median income, or $1,720 per month for an individual in 2004. Medicaid services subsidies are available to needs qualified individuals with incomes at or less than 300% of the federal SSI benefit, or $1,692 per month, and assets below $2,000. The 45-unit project includes 34 studio apartments and 11 one-bedroom apartments. All units are designated as Medicaid-eligible; but residents with eligible incomes for the rental programs who have too many assets to qualify for Medicaid may pay privately for services until (and if) they spend down their assets to within Medicaid limits.

State Lessons. The Coming Home Program partnership between the sponsor, key employees at the Division of Aging and Adult Services, the state Housing Finance Agency, the Office of Long-Term Care, and NCBDC lead to the successful adoption of assisted living regulations and an assisted living Medicaid waiver program. The combination of a supportive regulatory and Medicaid environment, together with access to pre-development lending, tax credits, and development technical assistance has resulted in one operating demonstration, three funded demonstrations, and 10 other projects in early or mid-stage development. The availability of appropriate and comprehensive technical assistance can help recruit and support projects in rural locations with committed, but not necessarily experienced, sponsors.

Florida Coming Home Program

Needs and Goals. Florida has the fourth highest number of people aged 65 and older in the United States (AARP, 2002). Of persons aged 70 and older, 29% require assistance with at least one activity of daily living; half earn less than $16,000 annually, and one-fourth report an average income of $6,410 (Reynolds-Scanlon, Reynolds, Peek, Polivka & Peek, 1999). As in most states, the default LTC option for a low-income older person with a disability is a nursing home. This is partially due to the lack of high quality affordable assisted living projects willing to serve Medicaid-eligible residents at the state's Medicaid reimbursement levels.

As the Coming Home Program grant applicant, the Florida Department of Elder Affairs listed three program goals: (1) establish a formal collaboration between partners to develop affordable assisted living projects focused on serving Medicaid eligible individuals; (2) develop a web-based clearinghouse of information, including best practices and development resources; and, (3) create private/public partnerships and advocacy to facilitate affordable assisted living.

Partnerships. The state agencies involved in the Florida Coming Home Project include the Department of Elder Affairs, the Florida Housing Finance Corporation (the state housing finance authority), and the Agency for Healthcare Administration (the regulatory agency for both assisted living and Medicaid). In addition, the state Coming Home Program officers organized a Committee on Affordable Assisted Living Facilities, consisting of housing, and service providers, regulators, policymakers, researchers, and provider associations.

Initial Challenges and Successes. The road to developing affordable assisted living in Florida started with overcoming several barriers. From the perspective of developers and operators, challenges included a wide range of state agencies with differing requirements, difficulty assessing the "market" due to the lack of a registry or standard definition of affordable assisted living, low Medicaid payments for services (which provided no financial incentives to providers), and limited assisted living experience among consultants familiar with the state's affordable housing programs. The state also identified additional barriers, including:

1. the lack of coordination between the state Medicaid agency, the assisted living licensing unit, the Department of Elder Affairs, the state's Housing Finance Agency, and non-profit developers; and,
2. the lack of commitment from the Florida Housing Finance Corporation (FHFC) to fund assisted living.

While the state has not been able to increase its service subsidies for assisted living during the Coming Home Program due to the state's budget crisis, Coming Home Program staff have been able to overcome the other challenges through the partnerships and the availability of technical assistance. Coordination and conflicts between state programs have been greatly reduced through formal and informal relationship building by state Coming Home Program staff. The state agencies involved in assisted living now work together on policy initiatives under the Coming Home Program and make themselves readily available to address issues encountered by the demonstration projects. The FHFC is testing a lending program for assisted living through a one time loan program and has also made pre-development lending available to demonstration projects. State and NCBDC staff have worked to provide training and direct technical assistance to overcome the gap in local consultants experience with assisted living's complex blend of housing and service programs as well as market assessment. This technical assistance has started the knowledge transfer process. These program accomplishments have encouraged mission-driven non-profits, those willing to work with the existing reimbursement, to undertake development projects to expand the availability of affordable assisted living resources in the state.

Demonstration Project. State Coming Home Program staff worked closely with the state public housing association to recruit public housing demonstration sponsors. The Pinellas County Housing Authority (PCHA) understood the need in their community and agreed to become a Coming Home Program demonstration. To create their affordable assisted living project, PCHA demolished an aging apartment and replaced it with Helen Piloneo Assisted Living, a 110-unit, 100%

affordable, assisted living project. The PCHA Commission approved issuing bonds to support the redevelopment. Operations are funded through Florida's Assisted Living for the Elderly (ALE) Medicaid waiver (1915c), Assistive Care Services (a state plan for adults with disabilities who receive SSI and need 24-hour unscheduled assistance), Optional State Supplementation (state supplement to adults with disabilities who receive SSI), and HUD public housing operating subsidies. The PCHA contracted with MIA Management Consultants to provide the services. MIA Management Consultants is focused on working with public housing agencies to develop affordable assisted living programs.

State Lessons. Even with low Medicaid rates, mission driven organizations are willing to take on the challenge of affordable assisted living when they have the support of the state. The Florida Coming Home Program's interagency coordination and individualized assistance has given projects the confidence to move forward. Providing subsidized lending programs for pre-development and permanent financing allows projects to move forward rapidly. Currently, three demonstration projects are operating, two will start construction soon, four are well into their development, and three more are in early stages of development. In addition, the successes have encouraged other groups to move forward. Several other community groups have responded to recruiting efforts, recognizing that in the absence of a willing, experienced non-profit organization community leaders will have to lead the effort to bring affordable assisted living resources to their community. State staff have recognized the continuing need for technical assistance, outreach to mission driven organizations, and consultant development to meet the challenges of producing new affordable assisted living resources within the constraints of Florida's Medicaid environment.

Vermont Coming Home Program

Needs and Goals. The Vermont HUD office published a Consolidated Plan for 2000-2004 that indicated a need for at least 2,000 units of affordable senior housing. The plan, based on a state survey, indicated that much of the existing affordable housing for older persons lacked support services and that a reduction in number of residential care units and a caregiver shortage would contribute to the need. Nationally, Vermont has the highest percentage of people aged 65 and older residing in a rural community. In addition, nearly 13% of Vermonters aged 65 and older are at or below the poverty level (AARP, 2002).

To address parts of their housing and services challenge, Vermont's Coming Home Program goals included supporting four demonstration projects, implementing assisted living regulations that support high service affordable assisted living, creating an unlicensed assisted living model to facilitate creative operations and financing approaches, identifying real costs for assisted living, creating appropriate reimbursement rates, exploring additional public subsidies, and building technical expertise on affordable assisted living within the affordable housing and service communities in Vermont to foster replication.

Partnerships. To respond to the Coming Home Program request for proposals, Vermont organized an affordable assisted living roundtable. The participants were the Cathedral Square Corporation (a non-profit developer and manager of affordable senior housing), the Department of Social Welfare (DSW), the Vermont Housing Finance Authority (VHFA), the Agency of Human Services, and the Department of Aging & Disabilities (DA&D). The agencies agreed to form a standing work group for the grant that would include representatives from demonstration projects as they were identified. DA&D received the Coming Home Program grant with VHFA and DSW as partners.

Initial Challenges and Successes. At the time of the state's Coming Home Program application, a variety of challenges existed in Vermont, including:

1. the lack of state regulations for high service assisted living programs (A regulatory drafting process was underway but was blocked in 1998, forcing DA&D to withdraw the proposed regulations and respond to concerns raised by a group of developers and residential care home operators.);
2. the lack of an adequate reimbursement program for individuals below a nursing home level of need; and,
3. the lack of a viable, small-scale assisted living model to respond to Vermont's rural community needs and preferences (e.g., 20 or fewer private occupancy units).

These obstacles had prevented even the most mission driven organization from trying to address the need for affordable assisted living in Vermont. Under the Coming Home Program, assisted living regulations were reworked with the assistance of the work group and were adopted in 2003, reimbursement levels were increased for residential care and assisted living models, and a small scale assisted living feasibility model is under development.

Demonstration Project. Cathedral Square is Vermont's first affordable assisted living residence, the first facility licensed under the new rules, and the first project to receive a HUD Assisted Living Conversion Program award. The building is a HUD 202 project that now has 80 units of independent living and 28 units of assisted living, of which 21 are affordable assisted living. Through an agreement with HUD, seven new independent living apartments were constructed next to the existing project with funding from other sources, including the Vermont Housing Conservation Board and federal special purpose funds. These seven units were built for market rate residents.

Cathedral Square Corporation (CSC) owns the building and provides the direct care services. Although it had previously provided limited social services, such as congregate meals, the assisted living program is CSC's entry into full-time personal and health service provision. The project was developed at the same time as the regulations and Medicaid program were in development. Project staff worked closely with the state to craft a regulatory and Medicaid program that supported the development of high quality, affordable programs.

State Lessons. Developing affordable assisted living required technical expertise that was not initially available in the state. The Coming Home Program allowed Vermont to facilitate collaborative partnerships, including workshops with experts that resulted in a transfer of knowledge from national experts to agency and housing sponsors. NCBDC and Vermonter's Coming Home are currently developing a financial model for small projects to continue the knowledge transfer and provide organizations with a critical development tool. The model will also allow the state to understand the reimbursement levels required to support small scale, high service assisted living projects in rural communities. The technical assistance, policy work, and program enhancements created in Vermont have been effective in creating affordable assisted living resources, with one operational demonstration program and 11 demonstrations projects at various stages of development.

Washington Coming Home Program

Needs and Goals. Washington's Coming Home Program application, submitted by the Department of Social and Health Service's (DSHS) Aging and Disability Services Administration (ADS), identified a lack of affordable assisted living resources for persons with low-incomes. In 2002, the cost of assisted living in Washington State ranged from $2,500 per month in rural areas to $5,000 per month in urban areas, yet almost 600,000 Washingtonians aged 65 and older had annual incomes of less than $25,000. Despite the state's established and well-funded HCBS program, organizations were not developing programs to serve Medicaid eligible individuals.

ADS received the Coming Home Program award in 2001. The goals for Washington's Coming Home Program included developing at least two projects per year for the three years of the grant and identifying and reducing policy barriers.

Partnerships. ADS partnered with the Washington State Housing Finance Commission (WSHFC) and the Rural Community Assistance Corporation

(RCAC). Washington's Coming Home Program staff and RCAC (a technical assistance provider for Western states) provided free workshops in six geographic regions of the state for agencies that finance assisted living, developers, and housing sponsors. In addition to technical assistance on combining housing and LTC programs, the workshops, promoted networking among individuals and organizations.

Initial Challenges and Successes. ADS identified the lack of affordable real estate development experience, including familiarity with assisted living, as a major obstacle to non-profit and rural providers. Lack of expert consultants for development and operations, was common. WSHFC's interpretation of LIHTC regulations, including concerns that the level of nursing services available in assisted living conflict with LIHTC guidelines, limited financing options. DSHS noted particular barriers to developing small, rural facilities, including the lack of economies of scale and organizations with the capacity to navigate the development process.

The Washington Coming Home Program addressed these challenges through three initiatives, the workshops described above, intensive project technical assistance, and inter-agency relationship building. The workshops were successful in developing technical resources by training developers on the state program, including the availability of the Coming Home pre-development loan. These developers, in turn, were able to introduce the project to their contacts. Several projects, including Quail Hollow (described below), resulted directly or indirectly from the workshops. The projects also successfully utilized the technical assistance provided by the state program staff and NCBDC to create feasible models. Economies of scale were introduced by partnering projects with existing service providers who could share staff and overhead cost across multiple programs. The economies of scale in the rural partnership model allow projects to support subsidized debt, allowing projects to overcome WSHFC's lack of funding by making them candidates for the Department of Agriculture's Rural Development loan program.

Demonstration Project. By national standards, Quail Hollow is a small facility, with only 16 apartments. Half of the 16 units are designated for individuals who qualify for the state's Medicaid HCBS waiver. The program sponsor is North East Washington Health Programs (NEWHP), a non-profit health care organization that provides medical, dental, home health, and hospice services and has a mission to provide medical services to individuals who lack health insurance.

The majority of project financing came from the USDA-Rural Housing Community Facilities Loan Program. This program provides direct loans at 4.5% (maximum 40 years amortization), is available to communities with populations of less than 20,000, and can be used to construct or improve facilities for health care and public services. While the USDA provided the low-interest loan, local health associations and the City of Chewelah worked together to make the project financially viable through donations of time and resources.

Economies of scale are achieved by sharing administrative and clinical staff with other NEWHP operations and by utilizing their bulk purchasing arrangements. The universal worker concept is also fully implemented. All employees are trained to do a variety of tasks, including personal care, housekeeping, and ordering food to maximize the efficient use of staff time. The Quail Hollow administrator explained that this flexibility saved the program money and allowed staff to respond to needs as they arise. For example, kitchen costs are minimized by getting everyone involved–day staff place and receive bulk food orders, the administrator buys additional products at a discount food chain, and night staff members provide additional grocery shopping as needed.

State Lessons. One of the earliest goals in Washington included attracting non-profit sponsors to develop affordable assisted living. Originally the state Coming Home Program manager attempted to attract sponsors through a Request for Proposals and by making presentations to existing operators of assisted living, but these approaches did not generate interest. The most successful activities for attracting and educating sponsors included conducting six one-day workshops, promoting the program via print and radio advertisements, and building capacity with existing developers who could then promote the program and provide technical assistance to other demonstrations. Individualized technical assistance to developers and project sponsors included real estate development, accessing public programs, regulatory requirements, and operational considerations. Additionally, state program staff facilitated the resolution of obstacles encountered by demonstration projects as they combined state programs.

Access to a $100,000 predevelopment loan, including its capacity to pay a portion of the developer fees, was a strong incentive for consultants to bring potential projects to the state project officer for consideration. Working with existing organizations with a track record in providing medical services to low-income individuals has benefited several projects. These strategies and lesson have resulted in three operational 16-unit rural facilities, five projects in the late stage of development, and two others that are in early pre-development.

LESSONS LEARNED

Following are some of the lessons learned from the first twelve years of the Coming Home Program. The first set includes those related to developing policies that promote the development of affordable assisted living. The second set includes lessons about how policies and programs need to be implemented to avoid unintentional obstacles to development and operations. Many of the state Coming Home programs will continue developing demonstration projects through 2005, when a final evaluation of the entire program will be produced that will include full policy and program findings and recommendations.

Policy Lessons

1. *Sufficient subsidy programs need to be available for the real estate and services portions of assisted living.* Single source capital grants or subsidized loan programs greatly expedite the creation of affordable assisted living. The more programs that have to be layered together to create affordable projects and the more competitive those programs are, the smaller the pool of organizations willing or able to take on the challenge will be.

2. *Cross agency partnerships are critical to the success of affordable assisted living.* Due to the complex and often conflicting requirements of the multiple programs that regulate and subsidize assisted living projects, agencies need to work together to eliminate barriers while allowing state objectives to be achieved. Coming Home Program states with fully committed and effective cross-agency partnerships have had better success in moving initiatives forward.

3. *Pre-development loan programs are critical to encourage and enable mission-driven organizations to pursue an assisted living project.* Without access to capital and a risk sharing arrangement with the lender, many communities do not have access to the funds required to explore a project. Even where organizations have the required capital, they are often unwilling to risk it on a project with so many uncertainties. The availability of the Coming Home pre-development loan program, as well as similar state programs, has been credited by several of the states as essential to their success.

4. *Technical assistance and outreach by state agencies to community organizations achieves significant results.* Community organizations need expert state assistance to understand the complex regulatory and subsidy systems and, equally important, to know they have an advocate within the state system. Many demonstration programs indicated that they would not have undertaken an affordable assisted living project without knowing that they had state staff members to assist them when they ran into obstacles. Demonstration programs identified state staff as particularly helpful in resolving slow state response times, program conflicts, conflicting information, and obtaining interpretations and clarifications.

5. *Expert assistance from development and operations consultants is critical to moving demonstration projects forward.* Mission-driven organizations willing to take on challenging and low-margin projects often lack expertise in one or more areas of development, finance, and operations. The combination of initial, grant-funded technical assistance from NCBDC, followed by in-depth technical assistance from project consultants funded through the program's pre-development loan, provided demonstration organizations with the technical capacity to explore projects. The Coming Home Program's continued role as an advisor throughout the development process provided demonstration organizations with an expert advisor to help them evaluate recommendations and options provided by consultants. Many of the demonstration projects identified the availability of expert consultants combined with access to Coming Home staff as an important factor in their decision to move forward.

6. *Cost data showing the per capita savings states obtain from implementing or expanding affordable assisted living is a powerful tool in policy debates.* The Coming Home Program found that federal and state programs save an average of 58% when a nursing home eligible Medicaid recipient is served in affordable assisted living.[3,4]

7. *The concern that large numbers of eligible recipients will "come out of the woodwork" and overwhelm the system if attractive alternatives to nursing homes are available still prevent some states from implementing large-scale assisted living programs.*

8. *Low state reimbursements for assisted living often limit the interest of high quality providers to only the most mission-driven.* To develop new, high quality affordable assisted living resources in states where rates cannot be raised, the specific needs of mission-driven organizations willing to operate affordable assisted living at cost need to be identified and addressed. Programs to encourage and support these organizations are critical to increasing supply.

Program Lessons

Just as it is important to create policies and programs that foster the development of affordable community-based options, it is vital to implement these policies and programs in a way that does not create new barriers.

1. *State programs need to operate efficiently and in a cooperative manner.* Some of the Coming Home Program demonstrations were hampered by slow Medicaid eligibility determinations, slow payments, insufficient payments, delayed licensing processes, adversarial survey agencies, and disinterested or unapproachable finance agencies. Once state policy and program problems become widely known, other organizations are unwilling to consider developing an affordable assisted living project.

2. *Service and real estate subsidies may present barriers even when they are in place and well funded.* Subsidy program design may present as much of a barrier to creating affordable assisted living as the absence of the program. For example, if complex affordable assisted living deals must compete with simpler, independent housing projects for funding and investors, they usually do not do well. The LIHTC program does not work well with rural (or any small) projects due to investor and underwriters' preference for large deals that spread their fixed costs over large transactions. State Coming Home Programs that created incentives in their real estate and service programs for affordable assisted living programs had the greatest success in creating new affordable assisted living resources.

3. *State program personnel need to be readily accessible to solve problems and creatively address obstacles identified by affordable assisted living projects.* One way to ensure this is to provide sufficient staffing and include project facilitation in staff evaluations. Coming Home demonstration project sponsors had the best access to state staff for problem solving when the staff's evaluations included producing affordable assisted living projects. State Coming Home Programs that included full time staff in both their project work plan and budget were best able to provide the time required to identify policy and program issues, coordinate cross-agency problem solving, develop initiatives, assist demonstrations, and manage the program toward its goals.

4. *State agency personnel need access to persons in authority to provide flexible and rapid solutions to program problems in order to keep project sponsors involved in the effort.* Coming Home Programs staffed by high-level agency personnel, or with the active support and involvement of high-level staff, were best able to move difficult issues to resolution.

5. *Access to experts for technical assistance on combining housing and service policies is critical for state policymakers and program administrators in their efforts to identify and solve barriers to affordable assisted living.* Several Coming Home states felt that without access to this specialized consulting they would have been unable to craft successful programs and solutions.

Suggestions for Future Research

The Coming Home Program demonstrated that assisted living can be created as a viable alternative to institutional LTC for persons with incomes as low as the federal SSI payment. Although there are regulatory and financial obstacles, these can be overcome through partnerships and joint programs among relevant state agencies and project sponsors.

While the Coming Home Program was able to devise practical solutions to barriers in each program state, partners in the program often had to improvise because information that could have guided decisions did not exist. Below are suggestions for future research that could help states refine their programs and better support organizations interested in developing affordable assisted living.[5]

1. *Reimbursement Rates:* States lack a reliable method for establishing Medicaid reimbursement rates for assisted living designed to attract good quality providers. This often results in insufficient or inappropriate incentives to develop or operate affordable facilities. Poorly constructed rates can also provide inappropriate incentives for providers to discharge or retain residents. Reliable methods for setting reimbursement rates need to be researched, developed, and documented to guide state programs. Appropriately designed rates would spur development of affordable assisted living, help states allocate scarce resources more effectively, and better achieve states policy and program goals for assisted living.

2. *Comparative Cost Analyses:* Although the daily reimbursement rate for assisted living is typically much less than for nursing facilities, state Medicaid and budget staff are uncertain whether committing dollars to assisted living actually decreases total LTC costs. To provide states with the information required for critical budget decisions, research is needed on the total per person cost for state and federal programs depending on where a person receives services (e.g., at home, in an assisted living or other residential facility, or a nursing home). Research is also needed to identify whether people are more likely to enter the state's Medicaid program to obtain assisted living versus nursing home services and at what rate.

3. *Non-Traditional Organizations' Role in Affordable Assisted Living Resource Development:* The potential for non-traditional community organizations, meaning organizations not currently involved in housing or services, to become sponsors of affordable assisted living is largely undocumented. Understanding their potential is important because traditional housing or service organizations do not always exist in communities with a need for affordable assisted living. Even where a housing or service organization does serve the area, they often do not have any interest in providing affordable assisted living or working with very low-income individuals. It would be helpful to know the interest, capacity, and needs of non-traditional organizations so that states could make better decisions about program design, support, and funding.

4. *Resource Needs for Organizations Developing Affordable Assisted Living:* Facilitating the development of affordable assisted living demonstrations was a requirement of the Coming Home Program. Some of the organizations assisted by the states succeeded in their efforts, and other, equally mission-driven groups (in the same states) did not. Research on why some organizations succeed and others do not would help states better understand what they need to do to modify their current programs to help more committed organizations to succeed.

NOTES

1. Illinois, Colorado, Oregon, and Arkansas.

2. The states awarded grants under Phase II of the Coming Home Program are Alaska, Arkansas, Florida, Iowa, Maine, Massachusetts, Vermont, Washington, and Wisconsin. RWJF and NCBDC published a Call for Proposals resulting in letters of intent from 29 states and full proposals from 13. Eligibility criteria included organizational capacity, demographic profile and need, cooperative ventures, state agency support, existing health care services, and financial viability. A National Advisory Committee reviewed the applications and recommended the list of final awardees. For more information, see *<www.rwjf.org/reports/nreports/cominghomee.htm>* or*<www.ncbdc.org>*.

3. Derived from NCBDC 2003 data for AK, AR, FL, IA, ME, MA, WA, and WI. VT did not have data available for this comparison.

4. Based on state and federal Medicaid payments, federal SSI, and state supplemental SSI payments.

5. The definition of assisted living promulgated by each state must be considered in this or any research in this setting.

REFERENCES

AARP. (2002). Across the States 2002: *Profiles of Long-Term Care*. [Report]. Washington, DC: AARP.

Commission on Affordable Housing and Health Facility Needs for Seniors in the 21st Century. (2002). *A Quiet Crisis in America*. [Report to Congress.] Washington, DC: Commission on Affordable Housing and Health Facility Needs. Available: *http://www.seniorscommission.org*

Metlife. (2003). *The MetLife Market Survey of Assisted Living Costs*. New York, NY: Metropolitan Life Insurance Company. Available: *http://www.metlife.com/WPSAssets/16670870001065792597V1F2003%20Assisted%20Living%20Survey.pdf* [Accessed 4/09/04].

Reynolds-Scanlon, S., Reynolds, S.L., Peek, M.K., Polivka, L., & Peek, C. (1999). *Profile of Older Floridians*. Tampa, FL: Florida Policy Exchange Center, University of South Florida.

Rogers, C.C. (1999). *Changes in the Older Population and Implications for Rural Areas*. [Report #90]. Washington, DC: U.S. Dept of Agriculture, Food and Rural Economics Division.

Index

AAAs (Area Agencies on Aging),
17-20,84-109,116-135
AARP (American Association of
Retired Persons), 15, 82-88,
140-159,170-171,190-193
Accessible Space, Inc., 47
Activities of daily living
(ADL)-related issues, 16-17,
30,60,140-145,173-174
ADA (Americans with Disabilities
Act), 29-30,116,128-129
Adams, L., 47
ADED (Arkansas Department of
Economic Development),
122-123
Adequateness-related issues, 54-56,
66-69
ADFA (Arkansas Development
Finance Authority), 122-123
ADL (activities of daily living)-related
issues, 16-17,30,60, 140-145,
173-174
Administration on Aging (AoA), 8,24-27
Admission risks (nursing home),
138-148
Advisory and planning agency
partners, 113
Affordable, Accessible Housing for
Arkansas With and Without
Disabilities program,
116-135
Agency partners, 113
Aging in place concept, 56-57
Ahrens, J., 1-4
Alaska-based initiatives, 40-49
ALCP (Assisted Living Conversion
Program), 21-23,30-36,68

Alley, D., 5-49
American Association of Retired
Persons (AARP), 15,82-88,
140-159,170-171,190-193
American Association of Service
Coordinators, 48
American Communities Survey,
139-159
American House, 45-48
American Seniors Housing
Association, 18,22
Americans with Disabilities Act
(ADA), 29-30, 116, 128-129
AoA (Administration on Aging), 8,
24-27
Apartment Finder, 128-129
ARC of Arkansas, 116-135
Area Agencies on Aging (AAAs),
17-20,84-109,116-135
Arkansas Department of Economic
Development (ADED),
122-123
Arkansas Development Finance
Authority (ADFA), 122-123
Arkansas Office of Long-Term Care,
187-188
Arkansas-based initiatives, 40-49,
115-136,180-200. *See also*
Public policy initiatives
Assisted Living Conversion Program
(ALCP), 21-23,30-36,68
Atkinson, P., 47

Bethany Homes, 49
Bibliographies. *See* Reference
resources

BOOK ORDER FORM!

Order a copy of this book with this form or online at:
http://www.haworthpress.com/store/product.asp?sku=5496

Linking Housing and Services for Older Adults
Obstacles, Options, and Opportunities

____ in softbound at $39.95 (ISBN: 0-7890-2779-8)
____ in hardbound at $59.95 (ISBN: 0-7890-2778-X)

COST OF BOOKS _____

POSTAGE & HANDLING _____
US: $4.00 for first book & $1.50
for each additional book
Outside US: $5.00 for first book
& $2.00 for each additional book.

SUBTOTAL _____

In Canada: add 7% GST. _____

STATE TAX _____
CA, IL, IN, MN, NJ, NY, OH & SD residents
please add appropriate local sales tax.

FINAL TOTAL _____
If paying in Canadian funds, convert
using the current exchange rate,
UNESCO coupons welcome.

❏ BILL ME LATER:
Bill-me option is good on US/Canada/
Mexico orders only; not good to jobbers,
wholesalers, or subscription agencies.

❏ Signature _____

❏ Payment Enclosed: $ _____

❏ PLEASE CHARGE TO MY CREDIT CARD:
❏ Visa ❏ MasterCard ❏ AmEx ❏ Discover
❏ Diner's Club ❏ Eurocard ❏ JCB

Account # _____

Exp Date _____

Signature _____
(Prices in US dollars and subject to change without notice.)

PLEASE PRINT ALL INFORMATION OR ATTACH YOUR BUSINESS CARD
Name
Address
City   State/Province   Zip/Postal Code
Country
Tel   Fax
E-Mail

May we use your e-mail address for confirmations and other types of information? ❏ Yes ❏ No We appreciate receiving
your e-mail address. Haworth would like to e-mail special discount offers to you, as a preferred customer.
We will never share, rent, or exchange your e-mail address. We regard such actions as an invasion of your privacy.

Order From Your **Local Bookstore** or Directly From
The Haworth Press, Inc. 10 Alice Street, Binghamton, New York 13904-1580 • USA
Call Our toll-free number (1-800-429-6784) / Outside US/Canada: (607) 722-5857
Fax: 1-800-895-0582 / Outside US/Canada: (607) 771-0012
E-mail your order to us: orders@haworthpress.com

For orders outside US and Canada, you may wish to order through your local
sales representative, distributor, or bookseller.
For information, see http://haworthpress.com/distributors

(Discounts are available for individual orders in US and Canada only, not booksellers/distributors.)

Please photocopy this form for your personal use.
www.HaworthPress.com

BOF05